TABLE OF CONTENTS

© Copyright 2018 - All rights reserved.

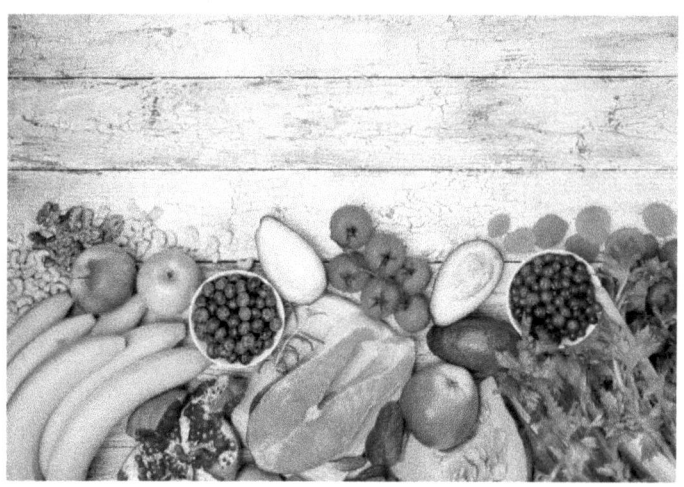

INTRODUCTION

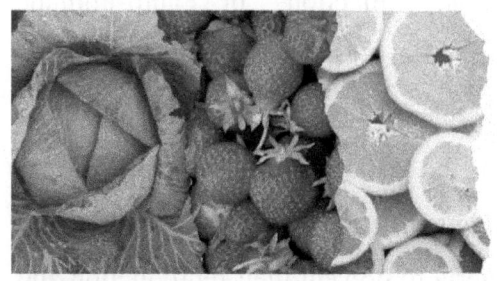

For those of you who have sprained your ankle and witnessed the associated swelling, warmth and pain will refer to the process as inflammation. But does the general public or the fitness instructors have a thorough understanding of this disease process?Inflammation is a very common part of our lexicon, we read about it in journals and articles and hear it mentioned on television.

Inflammation is the process the body uses to create an area of healing within the body. Whether it is as a result of injury or as a result of invasion by a foreign substance, it is the process which the body uses to protect itself. Inflammation is characterized by heat, swelling, redness and pain, but not all inflammation causes symptoms that we can sense or experience.

In scientific terms, Inflammation simply put a non-specific response to cell injury.An injury may occur due to trauma, infection or auto-immune responses.This complex process involves white blood cells, blood vessels and chemical mediators. The body relies on the inflammatory process for its protection. Inflammation destroys organisms such as viruses and bacteria to prevent their reproduction and propagation in our tissues. It also limits the tissue damage to a finite area and slows the spread of invading microbes. Inflammation is also responsible for clearing debris and making way for the repair of injured tissues and organs.

Toxins that the typical American is eating and drinking are the leading cause of the epidemic of an overweight population. Our bodies cannot handle a large number of toxins we consume on a daily basis. A good way to eliminate these toxins is to do the Anti-inflammatory diet cleanse or detox for the body. Do you think processed foods are toxin-free? The record has it that about 90 per cent of the money that Americans now spend on food goes to buy processed food.He reports that the flavour is replaced with chemicals to add flavor.To illustrate, there are approximately 350 different chemicals in high-quality artificial strawberry flavor.

Reducing this problem in your body is not a difficult task. To do this, you will need to watch what you eat and exercise regularly. When trying to avoid inflammation in your body; you will need to decrease your intake of processed food. All and any type of processed food will contain nutrition that increases the inflammation level in your body. Also, try to avoid foods that contain high amounts of sugar. Therefore, to prevent the problem you will need to eat vegetables and fruits.

To give the reader more than a perfunctory introduction to the topic, this book will focus basically on anti-inflammation methods and gestures to fight and get rid of inflammation in the body. It will also differentiate between acute and chronic inflammation, and also anti-inflammatory diet, foods that cause and fights inflammation.

Please, take a deep breath and enjoy the knowledge

that takes you through the journey to fight inflammation.

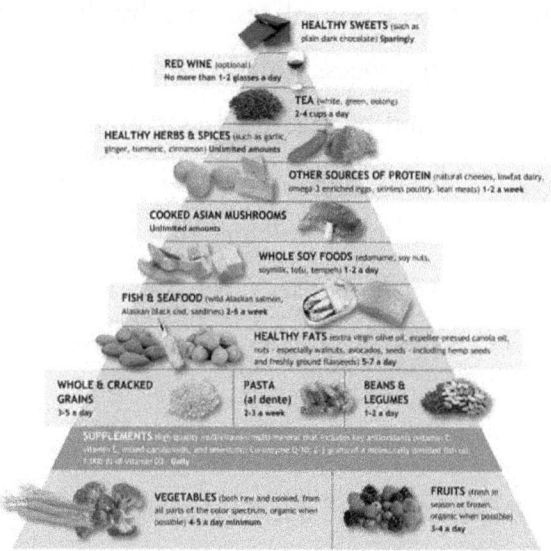

Pyramid Inflammatory Foods

CHAPTER:-1

BASIC KNOWLEDGE ON INFLAMMATION

Inflammation, the Body's First Line of Defense

Have you ever experienced red, painful, swelling, in a body part? This reaction in the body is called inflammation.

Inflammation is a normal response by the body to start the healing process. Inflammation can occur for many reasons and be classified as chronic or acute. Although the body regulates inflammation automatically, chronic inflammation can lead to a host of additional disease. Therefore inflammation should be closely monitored to make sure it doesn't persist longer than necessary.

Inflammation is the body's way of protecting itself against harmful stimuli such as pathogens, toxins or irritants. Acute inflammation is the initial response to injury or disease that appears within minutes or hours after entering the body. When acute inflammation occurs plasma and leukocytes (white blood cells) move to the area of injury — chemical reactions within the cells and tissue cause five distinct characteristics to appear. The five signs of inflammation are pain, redness, immobility, swelling and heat. As blood flow to the affected area increases, redness and heat appear. The more blood and fluid in the cells and tissues causes swelling. As the body releases chemicals, the nerve endings are stimulated which causes pain. Once the injurious stimuli have been removed, then inflammation and all of its symptoms will cease.

Acute inflammation has many causes such as physical injury, disease, toxins, chemicals and irritants. Burns, cuts, scrapes, scratches or broken bones all cause acute inflammation to occur quite rapidly within the body. Chemical irritants, toxins, and radiation depending upon exposure and hazardousness may cause instant inflammation or may appear over a longer period. Infections, pathogens, foreign bodies, viruses, bacteria and hypersensitivity may be delayed in showing signs of inflammation because they infect the body internally.

If inflammation persists because the stimuli cannot be removed then chronic inflammation will follow. Chronic inflammation can last for days, weeks, months or even years. It can also lead to a variety of inflammatory diseases such as hay fever, atherosclerosis, rheumatoid arthritis and cancer. Chronic inflammation produces a reaction in the body to simultaneously destroy and heal the tissue.

As a result, fibrosis occurs which causes collagen production and ultimately scar tissue formation. Chronic inflammation is a disease and should be treated immediately to avoid any further formation of wounds or disease.

In acute inflammation, resolution occurs throughout days. The tissue is restored to normal appearance after regeneration and healing are complete. Cellular blood flow returns to normal and white blood cells return to normal status within the body. Pain, redness welling should completely stop, and mobility should be completely restored. However in cases where chronic inflammation occurs, whether, from the start of from acute inflammation, a resolution can take longer and be more difficult. Cellular destruction, fibrosis, scar tissue and abscess formation are likely outcomes that can accompany chronic inflammation.Treatment of chronic inflammation involves medication, anti-inflammatories, changes in diet and exercise.

Chronic Inflammation: The New Science behind America's Deadliest Disease

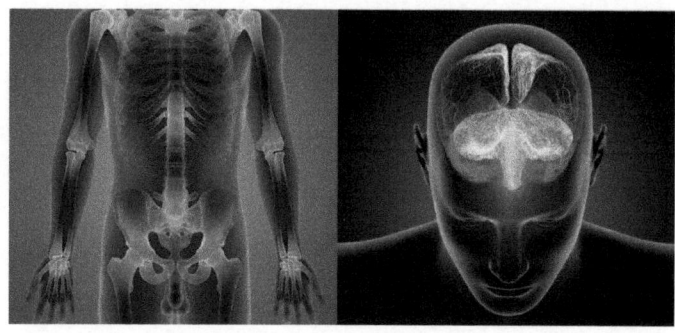

Inflammation is the body's natural response to injury or irritants. Inflammation should be treated so that people can get rid of it as soon as possible. If the inflammation gets chronic, it can damage heart valves and brain cells and can lead to diabetes by promoting resistance to insulin. It can also develop the deadliest disease called cancer.

Chronic inflammation is possibly well understood in its relation to cardiovascular disease because of the white blood cells rushing up to arteries as a result of cholesterol. This cholesterol causes damage to the arteries due to which a person experiences a heart attack or stroke.

Sometimes blood is also blocked in veins due to the presence of unwanted and unhealthy fats in the cells of arteries and capillaries in our body. Due to this fact, 75% of people in the USA suffer heart strokes in a calendar year. To overcome this fact it is important to burn fats that are unwanted in our body. They are deposited mainly due to our habitual eating of unhealthy food and snacks. It should be replaced with natural vitamins and mineral-rich diets like fruits and vegetables. It also cures all types of inflammation in our body.

Fat cells settle in the belly and around few organs, and this obesity also promotes inflammation. The fat cells churn out molecules which set inflammation in motion. If not treated on time, the inflammation becomes chronic due to which it can become deadly. According to the American Heart Association, a C-reactive protein lowers the risk of cardiovascular disease. So, all those people who want to save themselves from chronic inflammation should eat the right food on time. Still, there is little evidence to support any specific diet to protect against inflammation.

Cancer is the deadliest disease, and it is caused by many different processes and inflammation is one of them. Inflammation should be avoided by taking preventions and taking care of own self. Long-term effects that chronic inflammation has on our body and our health are the deadliest diseases which one can never dream of! The pain occurring due to the diseases is enough to kill a person, therefore; chronic inflammation is the new science behind America's deadliest disease.

Chronic inflammation makes a person bounded with nothing else but his or her pain in the body.The painful diseases do not let them live up their life with joy and prosperity. Chronic inflammation ultimately results in deadness. It also cannot be fully cured due to which it makes it difficult for a person suffering from it to be healthy and blissful in life.

In short, chronic inflammation is proved to be very harmful and deadly for a person. People should take very good care of them and avoid all those ways through which their lives can be at risk of chronic inflammation. There are scientists in America working over the cure of chronic inflammation, and they still didn't come up with the accurate cure of this deadly disease. So, preventions should be observed by people.

DISEASES OF CHRONIC INFLAMMATION

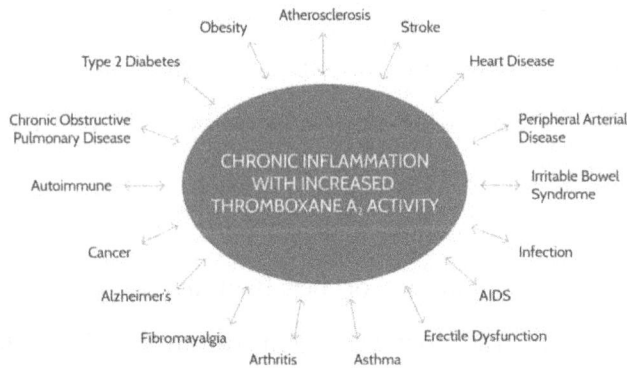

Chronic Inflammation Can Cause Serious Harm to Your Body

Inflammation touches many aspects of our life.It plays an important role in our body, and it's not something we can do without. But even as it protects us and plays a critical role when we are injured, it can cause problems if it gets out of control. When this happens, we refer to it as chronic inflammation.

It may seem a little strange that something so important to our well-being and good health can also ruin our health, and even cause death, but it is true. Chronic inflammation is something you want to avoid.

Heart disease and cancer have both been linked to problems with inflammation. About heart disease, it can cause coronary blockage and a heart attack. We've been told for years to keep our cholesterol low to avoid the buildup of plaque in our arteries, but scientist now believes that inflammation may play as important a role as cholesterol and plaque.

Inflammation is also a villain about cancer, particularly in the initiation of cancer. Things are not as clear here, and certainly, not all cancers are caused by inflammation. Nevertheless some of the cells and chemicals involved in inflammation have been shown to create mutations in DNA that can eventually lead to cancer; furthermore, it can also cause pre-cancer cells to become active cancer cells. A few of the cancers known to be associated with inflammation are colon, lung, stomach, oesophagus, and breast cancer.

Many other diseases are also associated with inflammation.Rheumatoid arthritis, osteoporosis, MS, lupus, emphysema, and gingivitis are all inflammation diseases. Indeed, any disease with a name with "it is" at the end of it is an inflammatory disease. A few examples are bursitis, tendonitis, arthritis, hepatitis, colitis, tonsillitis, and dermatitis.

- How Inflammation Begins and Proceeds
- Few of the several things that can initiate inflammation are:
- Infection by pathogens (bacteria, viruses and so on)
- Physical injury
- Foreign bodies that enter bodies such as splinters, dirt or other debris
- Chemical irritants

- Burns and frostbite

- Stress

- Toxins from air or water

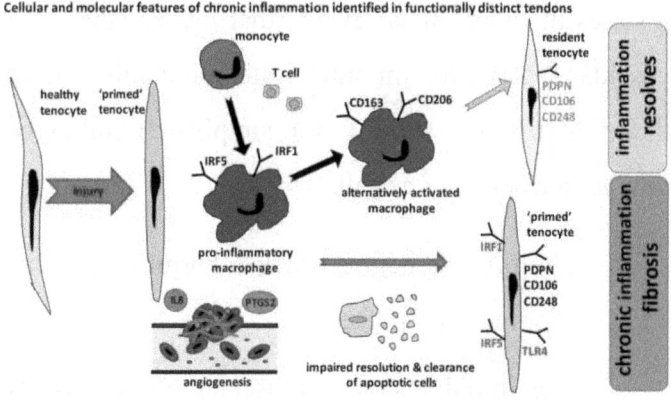

Cellular and molecular features of chronic inflammation identified in functionally distinct tendons

Everyone has experienced inflammation in one form or another. Its major symptoms are redness, swelling, heat and pain. In most cases, however, what we experience is acute inflammation.It is a short term process lasting only a few days to a few weeks, and in most cases, it ceases when the stimuli are removed. So for most people, it is not serious. Chronic inflammation, on the other hand, is inflammation that does not clear up properly.It persists for months, and sometimes, years and it can do considerable harm to your body.This aspect of this book is mainly concerned with chronic inflammation.

We'll begin, however, with an overview of acute inflammation. It goes through two main phases: a vascular phase and a cellular phase. And it consists of a series of biochemical events that involve the local vascular system, the immune system and cells within the injured tissue. A brief (and simplified) outline of how it takes place is as follows:

- The process begins when a harmful stimulus of some sort is detected.

- The initial response (vascular phase) comes from immune system cells present in the affected tissue. One of the major ones that detect it first and reacts is called macrophages. They have receptors that recognize pathogens and other foreign objects (not belonging to the body).

- These macrophages (and other particles) release inflammatory mediators that call in other particles. They also release mediator molecules, including histamine, that dilate the blood vessels in the vicinity. This increases the blood flow to the affected area; it also increases the permeability (leakage) of these vessels.

- The increased blood flow allows more infection-fighting immune cells to reach the area. It also increases the amount of glucose (sugar) and oxygen to the area to help nourish the cells. At the same time, the increased permeability of the vessels helps bring in plasma protein and fluids that contain antibodies and so on to the area.

- As a result of the above, the affected area swells and turns red. There is also some heating, and there may be a pain.

- The cellular phase begins as the increased size of the blood vessels helps the migration of white blood cells, mainly neutrophils and macrophages, into the area. They are particularly important when pathogens are present, in that they eat them, but they also perform other important roles such as assisting in the repair of the wound.

- One of the main things the above buildup does is "wall off" the area from further attack, particularly from bacteria and viruses.

- When the pathogen (or whatever) is overcome a cleanup of dead cells, and other debris begins. The initiation of a process where new, healthy cells replace the old ones begins, and soon the macrophages and other immune cells leave the area. And in the acute case, everything soon gets back to normal.

Chronic Inflammation

Unfortunately, everything doesn't always go as smoothly as described in the above process. Several things can go wrong, and when they do, serious problems can occur. (Thankfully, this doesn't happen too often.) The major problem is usually associated with the termination of the inflammation. In particular, the attack on the foreign objects doesn't stop as it should. Macrophages and other particles may be left behind, and they can do considerable damage to healthy tissue. One reason this might happen is that these particles check a "password" on the surface of cells and if it is a normal body cell they ignore it, but if it is foreign, they attack it. Sometimes, however, the password system breaks down, and the immune cells mistake body cells for intruders and destroy them. This leads to what is called autoimmune disease (such as lupus and MS).

In the same way, allergies of various types can occur when the immune system overacts. Pollens are usually considered harmless by the immune system, but in some cases, it can suddenly decide they are dangerous and attack them. The result may be asthma.

Or the immune system may see damage due to LDL cholesterol in the arteries as a problem and try to repair it. As a result, the immune cells become bloated and stick to the sides of the arteries creating plaque.

Most changes of this type occur when a person has a

weakened immune system so it it's easy to see why a strong immune system is important.

Who is Most at Risk

First of all, it's important to point out that everyone needs to be concerned about inflammation getting out of control, and everyone should do what they can to strengthen their immune system. Nevertheless, there are things that make some people more prone to chronic inflammation and other inflammation problems. They are:

Anyone who is overweight (in particular, obese). The immune system frequently mistakes fat deposits for intruders and attacks them. Also, fat cells can leak or break open; if this happens macrophages come in to clear up the debris, and they may release chemicals that cause problems.

- Anyone with diabetes. Studies show that diabetes II may be related to inflammation and that people with high levels of inflammation usually develop diabetes within a few years.

- Anyone with symptoms of heart disease or heart disease in the family. There are several relationships between heart disease and chronic inflammation. Also, it's well-known that the plaque in arteries, which results from inflammation, causes heart attacks.

- Anyone who feels tired and fatigued all the time. This is particularly important if no reason can be found for the problem. Fatigue is associated with inflammation.

- Anyone who works in a toxic environment. It's well known that toxins cause excess inflammation.

- Anyone suffering extensively from depression or anxiety. It's well-known that stress causes inflammation.

- Older People. Our body changes as we age and we tend to produce more pro-inflammation chemicals and fewer anti-inflammation chemicals.

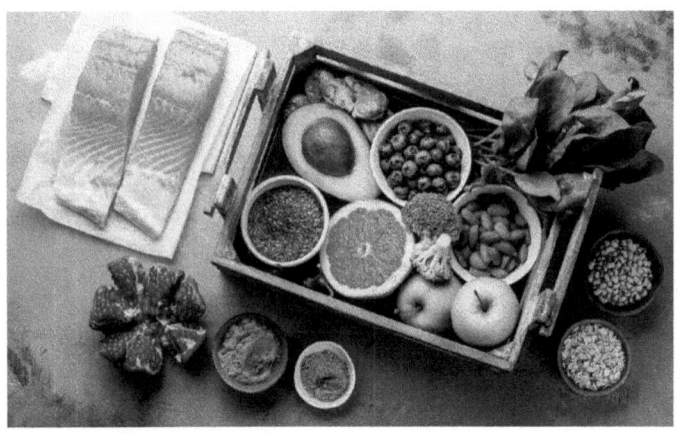

What You can do to Avoid Chronic Inflammation

The above list should give you a good idea what to do to avoid chronic inflammation. Nevertheless, I'll list some of the major things and briefly discuss them. I should mention, however, that genes play a role in whether or not you'll get chronic inflammation, and there's little we can do about them. A list of the major things is as follows:

- Eat a highly nutritious diet. It should include at least five servings of vegetables and fruit each day. Cruciferous vegetables are particularly important; they include broccoli, cauliflower, and cabbage. Other excellent vegetables are carrots, tomatoes, spinach and beans. Some of the best fruits are citrus fruits; berries such as blueberries and strawberries are also important. Other things that are particularly good are grains such as oats and whole wheat, nuts and seeds. Fish is also important as a source of omega-3, and you should eat it 2 to 3 times a week. At the same time, you should avoid simple carbohydrates, fast foods, soda, saturated fats and trans fat products.

- Don't overeat. Also, if you are over-weight, lose weight.

- Get sufficient sleep. For most adults 7 to 8 hours is sufficient.

- Exercise regularly. Exercise is, in fact, a good way to lower inflammation. Both aerobic and weights are important.

- Control your cholesterol, blood pressure and triglycerides.

- Avoid stress.

- Avoid toxins.

The Dangers of Chronic Inflammation

What would you consider a danger to your health? You were probably thinking about Heart attacks, strokes and cancer; right? Would it surprise you to know that one of the greatest threats to our health is chronic inflammation? All of us experience inflammation of one kind or another at some point in our lives; surely it cannot be very dangerous. Well, there are times where inflammation can be beneficial, and there are times that it can be harmful.

Inflammation is one of the bodies first responses to any kind of damage. If you were to cut your finger, bump your head or break an arm, within minutes, that whole area starts to swell and become a red. This is a process where the body's white blood cells, oxygen and chemicals are pumped to the wound, and the active inflammation protects us from infection and foreign substances such as bacteria. Once the white blood cells have done what was needed, and the wound starts to heal, the swelling then subsides.In some cases, the body's defence system triggers the inflammatory system's response when there are no foreign substances to fight off.Certain diseases can cause this to happen, and they are called autoimmune diseases.In this case, the body's immune system, which is meant to protect it, causes damage to healthy tissue.

Arthritis is a disease that is most commonly linked to chronic inflammation. The term arthritis is a general description of inflammation of the joints.However, not all types of arthritis are a result of inflammation. Inflammation of the joints can occur when an increased number of cells and inflammatory substances from within the joint cause irritation and wearing down of the cartilage. When enough damage has been caused, swelling occurs in the lining of the joints. The types of arthritis caused by inflammation include rheumatoid arthritis, shoulder tendinitis, gouty arthritis and Polymyalgia rheumatic.

Chronic inflammation can also have a detrimental impact on internal organs. Inflammation of the heart is known as myocarditis and can cause shortness of breath or swelling of one or both legs.Inflammation of the bronchial tubes located in the lungs, disrupt the absorption of oxygen and can lead to an asthma attack. Inflammation of the kidneys sustained over some time can lead to high blood pressure and eventually kidney failure.

A growing number of medical practitioners are starting to understand the consequences of chronic inflammation and the risk that it poses to human health. If doctors are now getting concerned, then surely we need to as well. We need to ask ourselves why we develop chronic inflammation and how we can prevent it. Did you know that information can cause premature aging? No amount of anti-aging creams or plastic surgeries will help if you cannot keep inflammation under control. The only way to do this is to take control of our health and ensure that we detoxify ourselves on a regular basis. It is only by keeping toxicity levels low that we can avoid chronic inflammation and premature aging.

Chronic and Acute Inflammation - Prevention and Treatment

Some of my patients have been asking me recently, about a new medical condition, inflammation, that's being investigated as the underlying cause of fatigue and most diseases including, cancer and heart disease. As I tell my patients, the truth is, inflammation is not something new, though our unhealthy diets and lifestyles may be adding to the rise in its occurrence. Inflammation, and its ill effect on health have been around for centuries, and have been well studied and treated by alternative, non-Western medicine, for just as long. It seems Western medicthe ine is just starting to catch on to damaging, chronic inflammation.

Inflammation, Friend or Foe?

Inflammation can help us and hurt us. Acute inflammation is the beneficial side of the condition that occurs when we injure ourselves through a cut, bruise, sprain or fracture. The surrounding area turns red and may become hot to touch. This is our immune system's first defence attempt at healing the damaged part. It sends white blood cells to the area which causes the tissues to heat up to kill an infection that may develop from the injury.

On the flip side, chronic, low-grade, ongoing inflammation, can be damaging to our overall health. Somehow, the body's immune system just keeps pumping out inflammatory responses, and instead of healing the body it starts to make it ill. But how does this happen? Well, it can come about from a variety of factors, the following being the most common:

- Smoking
- Too much alcohol
- Too much-refined sugar, high glycemic carbohydrates
- Insufficient good fatty acids (Omega 3's) in diet
- Insufficient antioxidants
- Too little exercise, overweight
- Diabetes

In short, the immune system starts to think of itself as under constant attack from poor diet and lifestyle habits and works overtime. Many researchers now believe that inflammation may be the key to understanding how all diseases start, from Alzheimer's, asthma, arthritis, GERD and ulcers, to heart disease and even cancer. Interestingly, treating these diseases successfully may also lie in treating the inflammation that's fueling them.

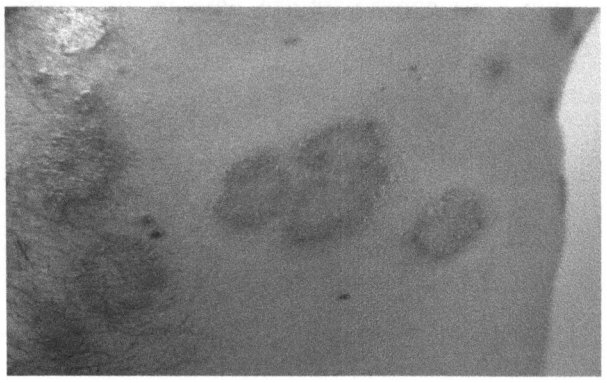

How Can You Get Rid of Inflammation?

To work on reducing inflammation, you first have to know if you have elevated levels of certain tests that are excellent markers for inflammation. These are: CRP - short for C-reactive protein, elevated in chronic inflammation.

Homocysteine - elevated, usually from a lack of folic acid and too high iron in the diet.

MPO - short for myeloperoxidase. A relatively new test for inflammation can help determine potential cardiac risk factors such as atherosclerosis.

Next, do everything possible to stop any inflammation-producing activities. For example, quit smoking, cut down on alcohol or limit it to special occasions. Get some exercise. People who exercise frequently tend to weigh less and have lower CRP, homocysteine and MPO levels. Reduce your weight as fat cells are filled with cytokines which boost inflammation. Get tested for diabetes. Untreated, uncontrolled diabetes can fuel inflammation, damage blood vessels, and put you at increased risk for heart disease.

Follow an inflammation-fighting diet such as the following:

- Limit sugar/refined carbohydrates. Cakes, pies, candy, some fruits, and high glycemic carbohydrates (bread, pasta), all create a high acid condition which fuels inflammation.

- Eat more good fats. Add high monounsaturated fats like mixed nuts, avocado, olive oil, as well as fatty fish like salmon, tuna, mackerel, sardines a few times a week. If you eat canned tuna, choose water-packed as the Omega-3's leach into the oil-packed varieties that will get drained off before eating. Or, take two 1,000 mg fish oil capsules a day.

- Limit acid foods. High acid foods like animal meats, eggs, lemon, grapefruit, and tomato.

- Eat more alkali foods. Yellow, dark green, vegetables like yams, kale, cucumbers fight inflammation by balancing acid with alkali.

- Add antioxidants. Our modern diet can't possibly contain enough antioxidants to do us much good fighting inflammation. Add a good supplement that contains Vitamin C, resveratrol, E, selenium, Vitamin D3, bilberry, blueberry. Spices like turmeric (curcumin), ginger, cayenne, parsley.

- Increase fiber. Fiber helps sweep inflammatory toxins out of your system.

- Avoid dehydration. Our bodies thrive on water to cool itself and dilute inflammatory acids. Drink at least ½ your weight in water a day.

What Are The Causes of Inflammation?

What Causes Inflammation at the Microscopic Level?

Microscopically, inflammation is made up of complex reactions that mostly involve the white blood cells, the blood vessels, and certain particles in the blood called plasma proteins. When an inflammatory stimulus is present, such as microbes, toxins, and lack of oxygen, the injured cells either release soluble factors into the blood or activate plasma proteins.These released agents are called inflammatory mediators. The inflammatory mediators then recruit different cells to the site of injury. Some of these cells, called phagocytes, phagocytose or eat the cause of injury and the injured cells. Other cells, such as leukocytes and endothelial cells help repair the injured tissues and promote wound healing.

What is the Difference between Acute and Chronic Inflammation?

Depending on what causes inflammation, the result can be acute or chronic. Acute inflammation is called such because it sets in rapidly, typically within minutes. It only lasts for hours to a few days. Its characteristic symptom is oedema or swelling, which is due to the oozing out of fluid and plasma proteins out of the blood vessels. When an acutely inflamed tissue is examined microscopically, the majority of the cells that can be seen are called neutrophils, which are big white blood cells.

Acute inflammation usually works, but sometimes, the invader or stimulus is not eliminated. The result is the progression of the inflammation to a chronic phase. Chronic inflammation may follow acute inflammation but may also be gradual and subtle. It lasts longer and is associated with the formation of new blood vessels, tissue destruction, and deposition of disorganized collagen called fibrosis. When chronically inflamed tissue is examined microscopically, instead of neutrophils, most of the cells that can be seen are lymphocytes, which are smaller white blood cells.

How are Inflammation and Disease Associated?

What causes inflammation can eventually lead to disease. When inflammation is not sufficiently controlled or becomes directed to the body's tissues, it becomes a mechanism of disease. It underlies many chronic diseases. These include cardiovascular diseases like atherosclerosis and coronary artery disease, rheumatoid arthritis, lung fibrosis, and allergic reactions. Inflammation also plays a role in Type 2 diabetes, cancer, and Alzheimer disease.

Due to the various diseases that can result from inflammation, inflammation is sometimes referred to as the "silent killer". This moniker has some merit since chronic diseases cause loss of normal functioning and in the long run, loss of life. In clinical medicine, a lot of attention is paid to controlling inflammation and preventing its damaging consequences.

CHAPTER:-2

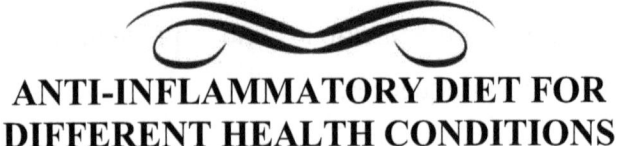

ANTI-INFLAMMATORY DIET FOR DIFFERENT HEALTH CONDITIONS

Who Needs an Anti-Inflammatory Diet?

Inflammation is often associated with injury. You stub your toe and the toe swells. This is the basic inflammatory reaction. Some people even understand that redness around a cut is also a form of inflammation that the immune system uses to heal the injury. What is not commonly known is the fact that inflammation occurs inside the body as well. When the body exists in an inflammatory state, the risk of illness, cancer and heart conditions can increase. An anti-inflammatory diet is an easy way to combat this aftereffect and reduce risk today.

"I Don't Suffer From Inflammation!"This is the most common statement and the least correct.Inflammation affects every person in the world at some point in their life. In western cultures, like the United States, a huge portion of the population is affected by inflammation every day. Being overweight or obese is the most common inflammatory condition. It is this inflammatory response that could be the cause of some weight-related conditions like diabetes. When fat cells grow, they take up the free space around the organs. Blood flow can be constricted, and the body often feels as though it needs to fight to function normally. When the body feels threatened, inflammation occurs as a natural, healing response. Unfortunately, unlike the small cut that will heal in a few, short days. Obesity takes time to correct and the longer the body lives inflamed, the greater the risk of long term effects. In the case of obesity, changing the diet by reducing calories will reduce body weight and thus reduce the inflammation in the body. This is the simplest benefit of an anti-inflammatory diet. However, people who are obese or overweight are not the only people who can benefit from an anti-inflammatory diet.

There are many illnesses and conditions caused by inflammation. These include asthma, arthritis, inflammatory bowel syndrome, pelvic inflammatory disease, endometriosis, diabetes, COPD, Psoriasis, Colitis, and Lupus – just to name a few.All-in-all, there are nearly 40 autoimmune conditions currently accepted by the medical community that are affected by inflammation.

What Can I Do?

The first step is to make dietary changes to reduce food based inflammation. Processed foods, fast foods and prepackaged foods can cause increased inflammation in the body. Replacing these foods with lean meats, whole grains and healthy fats will make a tremendous difference in how the body reacts to inflammation. Besides, if weight is a problem, reducing weight while changing to an anti-inflammatory diet can increase the benefits exponentially. Changing to an anti-inflammatory diet does not have to be in reaction to a disease or illness. Prevention is the best choice, and the anti-inflammatory diet can reduce the risk of contracting many of the listed illnesses. When the body feels as though it needs to fight for survival, inflammation occurs, so offering healthy foods that have an inflammatory effect is a great choice for all people including those who are young, healthy and feel they do not need an anti-inflammatory diet. Another great supplement to add to your diet is Nopalea.

Inflammation and Disease

There is a process in the body that is now believed by medical experts to be involved in all known disease processes from heart disease to cancer to Alzheimer's disease - inflammation. Most of you will have experienced inflammation before. Have you ever got a splinter in your finger? It got red and swollen, it may have bled a little, and it was certainly hot and painful - all the classic signs of inflammation. Now, inflammation is a normal response to an injury like this, and it serves us well. It helps to kill bacteria, parasites and viruses that try to invade us and this inflammation keep us healthy. This type of inflammation usually demonstrates a 100 fold increase in immune system markers, such as white blood cells and cytokines like IL-6, TNF alpha, or C reactive protein (CRP).

However there is another, the darker inflammatory response that happens in the body - what Dr Barry Sears calls "Silent Inflammation". This type of inflammation doesn't elicit the pain, swelling, redness and heat associated with classic inflammation and may only demonstrate a 4-5 fold increase in immune system markers - so can often be hard to detect. It can take years or even decades to develop and slowly but surely damages DNA and leads to disease. Unfortunately, modern medicine is not very good at treating this type of silent inflammation. It is the result of poor lifestyle choices and changing lifestyle and nutrition is a much better tactic than using anti-inflammatory drugs.

One of the primary sources of silent inflammation in the body is excess body fat. Fat is not just an unsightly inert substance that sits on your love handles or muffin top. It does not just serve as a reservoir of energy to be called upon when needed for energy. Fat is metabolic tissue that can cause all manner of things to happen in your body. Fat cells become infiltrated with high levels of immune cells that release inflammatory chemicals disrupting the uptake of sugar and burning of fat in liver cells contributing to insulin resistance, the onset of type 2 diabetes and narrowing arteries. Fat cells release chemicals that clot your blood, increase your blood pressure and convert inactive stress hormones into active stress hormones and contribute to conditions such as hypertension, stroke, cardiovascular disease and PCOS. (Take home point - lose body fat)

Here is a short inflammation questionnaire developed by Dr Barry Sears

- Are you overweight?

- Are you taking cholesterol medication?

- Are you taking blood pressure medications?

- Do you wake to feel groggy each day?

- Do you get carbohydrate cravings?

- Do you suffer from fatigue?

- Do you have brittle nails?

If you answered YES to 3 or more questions, you are

likely suffering from Silent Inflammation. In the aspect of this book, we are going to discuss inflammation as the cause of heart attacks (not cholesterol), inflammation and blood pressure, inflammation and cancer and inflammation and diabetes. I'll also discuss how to reduce inflammation through good nutrition.

Inflammation and heart disease

Now, this might be a little out there for some of you, especially as we have been brainwashed into thinking that saturated fat and cholesterol blocks arteries and causes heart attacks. But what researchers are now finding out is that inflammation is perhaps the major player here, not cholesterol.

As I mentioned the inflammatory response gets mobilised anytime, there is damage to the body. Unfortunately, the body is under constant low-level oxidative damage all the time from free radicals. These free radicals are nasty little unstable molecules that fly around stealing electrons from cells and generally causing havoc. The body's defence to these free radicals are antioxidants; antioxidants can safely donate their electrons to the free radicals rendering them safe. The main source of antioxidants in our body is formed from the food we eat, foods that contain amino acids and nutrients such as vitamin A, vitamin C, vitamin E, zinc, selenium and many other compounds such as alpha lipoic acid, green tea extract and carotenes.

The classic heart disease theory looks a little like this: Too much cholesterol in the diet causes cholesterol to be deposited in the arteries, such as the coronary arteries.

Cholesterol deposited in the coronary arteries causes narrowing or blocked arteries and hey presto a heart attack.

A novel approach to heart disease involving inflammation looks like this: A poor diet lacking in antioxidants leads to poor protection from free radicals and oxidative damage. As cholesterol travels through the arteries it moves in and out of the vascular epithelial cells. Cholesterol is attacked by free radicals and becomes damaged "oxidised cholesterol."Oxidised cholesterol is not recognised by the by the immune system which mounts an inflammatory reaction whereby immune cells called macrophages come along and eat the oxidised cholesterol.

The macrophage that has eaten the damaged cholesterol becomes a foam cell that is now trapped inside the epithelial cells that line the walls of the arteries.As these foam cells build up, they cause narrowing of the artery and can lead to reduced blood flow to the heart muscle. So cholesterol just seems to be the innocent bystander of the oxidative damage caused by a diet lacking antioxidants.

Inflammation and high blood pressure

Dr Barry Sears' "silent inflammation" not only contributes to heart disease but also to high blood pressure or what is sometimes referred to as hypertension. Now, hypertension is somewhat of a unique disease as there aren't any noticeable symptoms in the early stages, so it's a good idea to get your blood pressure checked and do all you can to keep it in the "normal" zone.

Many of you will have gone to the GP and had your blood pressure measured. You may have been told that your blood pressure is 120 over 80 or 135 over 90, but what do these numbers mean?

When your heart beats it forces blood out into the arteries, which produces the first number in a BP reading.This number should be 120mmHg, which is considered normal, any higher than 140mmHg would be considered bad. Conversely, if that number is too low, it can also be bad. However, if the arteries were not strong or did not produce some resistance against the pressure of the blood being pumped out by the heart, the arteries would rip open. This resistance produced by the arteries is the second number in a BP reading. This number should be 80mmHg, which is considered normal, any higher than 90mmHg would be considered bad. Conversely, if that number is too low, it can also be bad.

From scientific research, we can make estimations about your life expectancy based on your blood pressure, as you can see the higher your blood pressure, the shorter your life expectancy.

BP of 130/90 = 67 ½ years

BP of 140/95 = 62 ½ years

BP of 150/100 = 55 years

The arteries are not just static tubes through which the blood flows; they can constrict and dilate depending on different factors such as stress, smoking and nutritional status. If a tube through which a fluid is moving narrows, the pressure in that tube increases, conversely if it widens, the pressure in the tube decreases much like what happens in arteries.

Many of you will have heard that if you are overweight or eat too much salt, you will have higher blood pressure and that to reduce blood pressure you need to reduce salt in the diet - true, but this is not the only mechanism at work here. Inflammation also plays a big role in high blood pressure.

To understand this, we need to learn a little bit about vascular biology (I can see your eyes glazing over but bear with me). The arteries are lined with cells called endothelial cells that produce a host of chemicals that can constrict or dilate your arteries. One of the major vasodilators produced by endothelial cells is nitric oxide, Nitric oxide tells the arteries to relax and widen, which will reduce blood pressure. What we know is that C-reactive protein (CRP) that inflammatory cytokine that I mentioned earlier can decrease the production of endothelial nitric oxide and increase inflammatory nitric oxide, leading to vasoconstriction and increased blood pressure. Inflammation devours nitric oxide. We also know that oxidative damage and free radicals reduce nitric oxide and that hypertensive patients have reduced antioxidants such as glutathione, superoxide dismutase, vitamin E, vitamin C, vitamin A, copper, and polyunsaturated fats.

So there you have it - inflammation causes increased blood pressure.

One thing that has been shown to reduce blood pressure is something called the DASH (Dietary Approaches to Stop Hypertension) diet. The DASH diet is essentially a low salt, low carb diet that is higher in protein and essential fats.

- Meat poultry and oily fish 2-4 servings a day

- Vegetables 6-8 servings a day

- Fruits 4 servings a day

- Dried beans, seeds and nuts 1-2 servings a day

- Low-fat dairy products 1-2 servings a day

- Cereals, grains and pasta 1-2 servings a day

- Fats and oils 4-5 servings a day (mainly unsaturated fats like olive oil, fish oil, however some saturated fat is allowable)

- Fibre - 50g a day (mix of soluble and insoluble fibre - may need to use a fibre supplement)

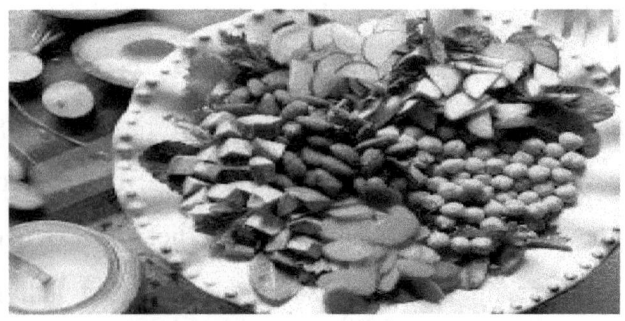

Again this diet is lower in inflammatory foods and higher in antioxidants much like the Mediterranean diet I mentioned earlier (in fact there are many similarities).

Inflammation and cancer

A growing number of cancer researchers are concluding that cancer is an inflammatory disease and that the longer there is inflammation present in a tissue or an organ, the higher the risk of associated carcinogenesis.

Epidemiological studies estimate that nearly 15 per cent of worldwide cancers are associated with microbial infection; this may include cervical cancer and the HPV1 virus, bowel cancer and inflammatory bowel disease due to bacterial dysbiosis and stomach cancer secondary to H. Pylori infection. All of these infectious agents are associated with an inflammatory response in the body.

One way the immune system deals with these invaders is to release free radicals that kill the invading viruses and bacteria. However, these free radicals can also damage the DNA of healthy cells. These cells either repair themselves or die. If a large number of cells in an area dies secondary to infection, there is an inflammatory mediated response that may lead to tumour growth.

Many other cancers may be the result of long term chronic irritation and inflammation such as smoking and lung cancer or chemical toxicity (xenoestrogens) and breast cancer. Once again there is DNA damage, inflammation cell death and tumour growth.

Eventually, these tumours are capable of releasing inflammatory chemicals that can maintain their growth, such as by initiating the growth of new blood vessels that feed tumour growth.

I'm not going to present an "anti-cancer" diet, but I am going to suggest that sugar could be a contributing cause to cancers. Cancer loves sugar is a statement that seems to get banded around. Cancer cells appear to use a combination of lots of sugar and specific proteins to ignore cellular instructions to die off and keep growing. Plus we know that people who consume more omega 3 fats, antioxidants and fibre suffer less from cancer. So by eating a diet that is anti-inflammatory such a diet rich in oily fish, fruits and vegetables may protect you from cancer.

Inflammation and diabetes

Inflammation might also be a cause for type 2 diabetes. This type of diabetes is generally considered to be the results of being overweight and from eating too much sugar which makes the cells resistant to the effects of insulin.

But what might be the cause is... inflammation!

I've already discussed how being overweight causes the release of a whole load of inflammatory chemicals that contribute to what Dr Barry Sears calls "silent inflammation". Well, research on mice shows that inflammation provoked by immune cells called macrophages (the same cells that become foam cells and lead to blocked arteries - and that are also concentrated in fat cells) leads to insulin resistance and type 2 diabetes.

This research was done in mice that were genetically engineered to lack a specific gene present in the insulin-producing cells of the pancreas. These genes are sensitive to the inflammatory response caused by macrophages, and when these mice lacked the gene, they did not develop diabetes, even when fed an extremely high-fat diet.

Now this research was done in mice and applying it to humans needs to be taken cautiously. However, there is a good argument to reduce inflammation to protect the pancreas.

Other anti-inflammatory foods that can be very useful in protecting yourself from "silent inflammation" include:

- Oily fish rich in omega three fats

- Ginger

- Garlic

- Turmeric

- Quercetin found in onions, broccoli, tea, wine and grapes.

Anti-Inflammatory Diet for Pain Relief

Most people are aware of the mechanical causes of

back pain such as ligament sprains, muscle, strains, slipped discs, etc. Fewer people are aware of inflammatory spinal pain, and the fact that our diets can lead to systemic inflammation that results in pain throughout the body. It's important to be knowledgeable about the ways diet can promote inflammation, the foods that cause it, and a list of foods that fight inflammation.

There's no doubt that we don't make great food choices as a country, as evidenced by the ever-increasing percentages of obesity and lifestyle diseases.The standard American diet now depends largely on "comfort foods" where typically 60% of the calories come from oils, flour and sugar.While these foods taste good, they contain a high amount of arachidonic acid.Why should you care about arachidonic acid?

Arachidonic Acid

The two common fatty acids in our diet are Omega-6 and Omega-3 fatty acids. It is recommended that we consume a 1:1 ratio of these fatty acids, but the average American diet can have as much as a 30:1 ratio. When our diet is high in omega-6 fatty acids, it shifts our tissue towards the pathogenesis of many diseases: proinflammatory, prothrombotic and constrictive. One form of Omega-6 is arachidonic acid. While this acid in small quantities is essential for proper nutrition, in high volumes it can promote excess inflammation throughout our bodies. The arachidonic acid that we eat is eventually converted into prostaglandins that can cause pain and inflammation. To a certain extent, we are eating pain and inflammation with poor dieting.

Food High in Omega-6: Omega-3 ratio

To reduce inflammation, it is recommended that you avoid foods that have a high ratio of Omega-6 to Omega-3. The following is a list of some common foods that tend to have a high ratio.

- Grains - 20:1

- Seed and seed oils - 70:1

- Soybean oil - 7:1

- Chicken - 15:1

- Potato Chips - 60:1

Benefits of Omega-3

The long-chain forms of Omega-3 fatty acids are DHA and EPA. DHA is the building block of brain tissue, and EPA is its precursor. The following is a list of the benefits and conditions that are improved with Omega-3 acids in the diet.

- Healthier, stronger bones

- Improved mood regulation

- Reduced risk of Parkinson's

- Reduced risk of death from ALL causes

- Prevention of vascular complications from Type-II diabetes

- Gallstones

- Multiple Sclerosis

- Brain and eye development in babies

- Peripheral artery disease

- Preventing postpartum depression

- Combating cancer

Foods High in Omega-3

- Flax seed oil

- Canola Oil

- Walnuts

- Fish

- Shellfish

- Krill

- Cod liver oil

- Omega-3 enriched eggs

- Pasture-raised meats

- Wild rice

- Beans

Anti-Inflammatory Foods

Along with focusing on foods that will provide the correct ratio of Omega-6 to Omega-3 fatty acids, there are also certain foods that have anti-inflammatory properties:

- Vegetables

- Fruit

- Sweet potatoes and other tubers

- Dark Chocolate

- Red wine

- Coffee and tea

- Ginger, turmeric, garlic and other spices

- Olive oil, Coconut oil and butter

A quality fish oil supplement needs to be in your diet. It's important to look for fish oil that has been molecularly distilled and contains at least 500mg of both DHA and EPA. There are plenty of fish oil supplements on the market that will advertise 1000mg of fish oil, but not all contain the recommended amount of those two acids.

An Anti-Inflammatory Diet for Leaky Gut Disease

Leaky gut disease or leaky gut syndrome is a condition that can be caused by antibiotics, infections, parasites, toxins, or poor diet. The significant feature of the condition is alteration or damage to the bowel lining. As the lining becomes more permeable than normal, it allows microbes, undigested food, waste, toxins, or large macromolecules to enter. Some researchers believe that these substances have a direct effect on the body; others think the problem is an immune reaction to those substances.

Whatever has caused it for you, you probably just wish the symptoms -- everything from acne and indigestion to anxiety and fatigue to joint pain and constipation, to name a few - would go away. Unfortunately, that wish can lead to treating just the symptoms. If you have Leaky Gut Disease, however, it's important that you don't just address the symptoms. You need to focus on the root causes of the condition.

One -- if not the main one -- of these root causes is diet. While practitioners disagree on a lot of things about Leaky Gut Disease (whether it even really exists, for example), the diet primarily recommended for those suffering from it - the anti-inflammatory diet - is generally acknowledged to be a healthy one for almost everyone.

The anti-inflammatory diet isn't a diet; it's more of an eating plan. And if you do a little research, you'll find that there's not just one anti-inflammatory diet; there are several, each with a different spin. For our purposes here, I've tried to present what is a "generic" version. This version does share with the others the concept that continued, and out-of-control inflammation leads to illness and that following an eating plan that avoids inflaming the body promotes health and can help prevent disease.

In general, an anti-inflammatory diet includes:

- Plenty of fruits and vegetables
- Plenty of whole grains (e.g., brown rice, bulgur wheat)
- Lean protein (e.g., chicken, fish)
- Anti-inflammatory spices (e.g., curry, ginger)

- Omega-3 fatty acids (such as those found in fish, fish oil supplements, and walnuts)

- A reduction in

- Refined carbohydrates (e,g., pasta, white rice)

- Red meat and full-fat dairy foods

- Saturated and trans fats

- No refined or processed foods

Many who endorse this diet also urge that you avoid refined sugar and products that contain it as well as caffeine and alcohol. And while drugs don't fall into the diet category, have your doctor review your prescriptions and monitor your use of OTC drugs, especially NSAIDS.

One word of caution regarding this plan: The effects you experience (i.e., an improvement in your symptoms) will not be as immediate as they would be if you treated yourself with medications. You probably need to give the anti-inflammatory diet at least two weeks versus the hour or two a medicine might take. On the other side, this diet might have a bonus effect not usually found in medications: weight loss!

The Role of Inflammation in Aching Joints and Injury

When you suffer from aching joints or sustain an injury, there is usually an accompanying inflammation that is noted as one of your symptoms. It is important to understand the different role inflammation can play following an injury or with aching joints such as tendonitis, bursitis and arthritis.

The Purpose of Inflammation

Inflammation is the body's reaction to damage. The tissue reacts to injury by swelling which in turn causes a soothing and stabilizing tightening. In the case of a cut or scrape, the swelling is designed to keep out bacteria. With a sprain or injury to joints and muscles, the swelling helps to stabilize the area and stop the joint in question from moving excessively in an attempt to protect it and allow it to heal. Inflammation helps to isolate an injured area as well as to help heal damaged tissue and protect openings from being invaded by foreign objects and bacteria.

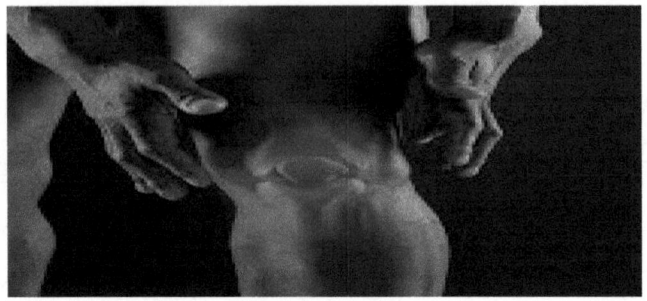

Perpetual Inflammation

Inflammation becomes troublesome because it can create further inflammation. This becomes very troublesome and continues to perpetuate further inflammation. This can be at the root of many aching joints and can also inhibit movement which in turn makes healing more difficult.

When Inflammation Heals

When you are suffering from inflammation, your doctor will investigate the cause before assuming the inflammation must be reduced. When inflammation is part of the healing process, it is not necessarily the best idea to try to reduce it. However, as inflammation progresses away from the healing process and towards creating scar tissue, it can begin to cause damage if the scar tissue itself does not heal. Interestingly, Neuroscientists at the Lerner Institute in Cleveland feel that the role inflammation plays in healing may be interrupted when attempts to decrease inflammation are made following injuries, especially those experienced by professional athletes. They believe inflammation heals injured tissue and that stopping inflammation may lead to further damage to the muscle.

Symptoms of acute inflammation are as follows:

- Pain
- Redness
- Immobility
- Swelling
- Heat

Inflammation and Aching Joints

Inflammation causes pain because of the swelling.

Swelling puts pressure on nerve endings which results in somatic pain when dealing with the musculoskeletal system. Joints, muscles, bones and tendons all suffer from somatic pain as a result of the swelling associated with inflammation. Aching joints are sensitive to stretch in the muscles as well as a lack of oxygen which can cause muscle cramps.

Treating Aching Joints and Inflammation

There are many known treatments for inflammation including acetaminophen and corticosteroids, as well as natural remedies such as devil's claw, hyssop, ginger and turmeric.

There are also many products available to aid in easing the pain of aching joints including:

- Kextin: Protects from cartilage destruction, douses inflammation and rebuilds your joints!

- Eazol Joint Pain Relief: FDA registered homoeopathic pain reliever

- Joint Relief Solution: Helps you move without pain and have more flexibility

- Natural Body Defense: Promotes healthy joint health and reduces inflammation naturally

- Juvamend: Relieves discomfort, improves flexibility, increases mobility and soothes your joints

- Joint Advance: Supports and maintains healthy joints and healthy mobility

It is best to see your doctor to identify the causes as well as to seek ways to ease the pain and discomfort of your aching joints.

The Benefits of an Anti-Inflammatory Diet

Inflammation is quickly becoming the next big medical discovery.People suffering from obesity have inflammation issues.Diabetes, arthritis and asthma are all associated with inflammation in the body.Not to mention the link to certain heart conditions and cancers. Reducing the inflammation in your body with an anti-inflammation diet can cause an immediate change to how you feel, not to mention the long term effects of the dietary change on health and well-being.

The first step to adopting an anti-inflammatory diet is to understand the effects of foods on the body. Food provides nutrients and vitamins the body needs to survive. The idea of eating to live not living to eat is a huge push for the weight loss community, but this idea should not just be followed when needing to lose a few pounds. Certain foods have high concentrations of anti-oxidants and natural anti-inflammatory nutrients that may reduce the effect of inflammation on the body.It is these foods that cornerstone the anti-inflammatory diet.

The Role of Omega 3 and Other Fatty Acids

Fatty acids are present in many foods that contain oil. The best natural source is fish like salmon and sardines.However, Omega 6 fatty acids are prevalent in western diets over Omega 3s. This is because commonly eaten foods like chicken, turkey, eggs, nuts and vegetable oils are rich in Omega 6 fatty acids. What people don't realize, however, is that these fatty acids need to be balanced with Omega 3s for optimal health and anti-inflammatory action.

Most western diets include ten times more Omega 6s than Omega 3s. Some diets include as much as 30 times more. The optimal ratio is four parts Omega 6 to every 1 part Omega 3.Increasing Omega 3 fatty acids in the diet can reduce inflammation in the body and thus reduce the effect of this condition on health and general well-being. Foods rich in Omega 3s include fish oil, kiwi, black raspberry and various nuts. The most readily available source of Omega 3s is flaxseeds. Many people mistake fish oils for the best source, but flaxseed oils tend to have the most readily available Omega 3s that make absorption in the body easier. Flaxseed oils contain about 55% ALA (alpha-linoleic acid) which is an Omega 3 fatty acid.

Fatty Meats Be Gone

Another simple change to reduce inflammation in the body is the reduction of fatty meats. Red meat is the worst of all meats for people suffering from inflammation. Choosing a leaner cut or a leaner alternative is a good option.Bison and venison are two options that tend to contain less fat. Grass-fed cows also have fewer inflammatory characteristics on the body. Fish, lean chicken, turkey, soybeans, tofu and soy milk, are all lean choices for decreasing inflammation. But some of these meats tend to be higher in Omega 6s. To combat the fatty acid imbalance that may be increasing inflammation, try cooking these meats in olive oil or adding flaxseed oil to the final dish to boost Omega 3s.

The Danger of Processed Foods

The worst food to eat when suffering from inflammation is a processed carbohydrate. These foods offer very little nutritional value and should be replaced with whole grain alternatives. All flour is wheat based, but processed flour is stripped of the healthy grain wholeness and bleached. What is left are empty calories sure to swell the body even more. Simply replacing white bread with whole grain bread and white flour with whole wheat flour that is unbleached can make a big difference in how your body reacts to your diet.Another great supplement to add to your diet is Nopalea.

CHAPTER:-3

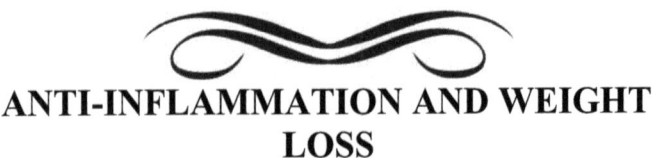

ANTI-INFLAMMATION AND WEIGHT LOSS

Inflammation and Weight Loss Resistance - Is This Connection Valid?

Contrary to popular belief, inflammation isn't just about headaches or swollen joints. It plays a part in everything from digestive disorders and depression to allergies, autoimmune diseases and abdominal fat. Surprisingly even more so, its very existence can greatly interfere with your fat loss goals.

So, you may be asking yourself, "What does fat loss have to do with inflammation?" or "Is inflammation and weight loss resistance connected?"

Quite simply, a lot and yes. First, inflammation has been shown to precede the development of both obesity and diabetes.These elevated levels of inflammation predict future weight gain and insulin resistance. Excessive or persistent inflammation leads to tissue destruction, disease and increases in weight (as well as an inability to lose weight). Therefore, reducing inflammation is an critical step in allowing the body to lose unwanted fat and achieve optimum health. Why? Because inflammation and weight loss resistance is a proven issue.

A little back story....We have fat-burning pathways in our liver and muscle cells that influence the interaction between our insulin sensitivity, inflammation and weight. An imbalance in these pathways contributes to inflammation, obesity and insulin resistance. Because of this interaction, anti-inflammatory supplements and lifestyle habits which increase our insulin sensitivity help to optimize our bodies' fat-burning capabilities and are also beneficial in the struggle against reaching and maintaining our ideal weight.

Here are a few suggestions to get your inflammation under control - and slim your waistline in the process.

- Improve your digestive health

- Get your immune system in check

- Eat more well-balanced, whole foods

- Add in systemic enzymes

- Take your omega oils

- Stabilize your blood sugars.

Believe it or not, you can address all the items above simply and easily, without turning your life upside down or depriving yourself. Yes, you can stop the vicious cycle of inflammation, weight loss resistance and weight gain that has tormented the majority of Americans for years and achieved the success you so desire. While chronic inflammation is a disease of modern times, it can easily be avoided with the right diet, supplements, and lifestyle factors. While that may seem overwhelming, it is quite simple. Keep reading...

Putting it all together What are the causes of inflammation? In a nutshell, our modern lifestyle.Specifically, dietary triggers (fructose, wheat and processed foods), environmental toxins, poor sleep, poor gut health and STRESS, all-cause inflammation on their own. When joined together, they are a volatile mix.

Lose Weight and Feel Great with the Anti-Inflammatory Diet

The anti-inflammatory diet can make you feel great! "How," you ask.By cutting out or significantly reducing your consumption of pro-inflammatory foods. When these foods are cut from your diet, inflammation in the body reduces taking stress and strain from the joints and organs.

While following this diet your chance of weight loss also goes up. "How does this happen," by reducing your consumption of grain and wheat products, sodas, and other simple sugars that cause excess weight.

I'll start this discussion by telling you what extra inflammation in the body causes; chronic pain, arthritis, fibromyalgia, chronic fatigue syndrome, allergies, acne, Alzheimer's disease, heart disease, cancer, hypertension, depression, and diabetes. However, this is a shortened list there are many other conditions out there caused by inflammation.

In summary, the fewer inflammatory foods we eat, the less inflammation we have in the body.

Background Information on Pro-Inflammatory Foods:

Grains, refined sugars, partial-hydrogenated oils, vegetable and seed oils are from modern man. These foods have been around a short time; hence, obesity and disease are on the rise.Humans are genetically adapted to eat fruits, veggies, nuts, lean meats, and fish, foods not related to chronic diseases.

Why Do Grains Inflame?

Grains contain a protein called gluten. Gluten is the main cause of many digestive diseases, such as celiac disease, also a contributor to frequent headaches. They also have a sugar-protein called lectins which has been shown to cause inflammation in the digestive system. Grains also contain phytic acid which is known to reduce the body's absorption of calcium, magnesium, iron, and zinc.

Lastly, grains contain high amounts of fatty acid

biochemicals called omega-6 fatty acids which do cause inflammation. Fatty acid biochemicals known as omega-3 fatty acids are anti-inflammatory and found in fresh fish and green vegetables.

Anti-inflammatory foods

- All fruits and vegetables (raw or lightly cooked)

- Red and sweet potatoes

- Anti-inflammatory omega-3 eggs

- Raw nuts

- Spices such as ginger, turmeric, garlic

- Organic butter, coconut oil, extra virgin olive oil

- Fresh fish, avoid farm raised

- Meat, chicken, eggs from grass-fed animals

- Wild game such as deer, elk, etc.

- Water, organic green tea, red wine, stout beer

How to Lose Weight by Reducing Your Body's Inflammation

If you've been researching how to lose weight and you haven't yet come across the science of chronic inflammation, then you're in for a surprise. There is so much information out there on diet and exercise, enough to scramble anyone's thoughts - and yet the hidden factor, lurking beneath the surface of weight problems, is chronic, underlying inflammation. Indeed, chronic inflammation is now considered to be the common factor in almost ALL diseases. Inflammation is a natural process, but when it becomes chronic, it's all wrong.

The reason this is so vital to understanding is that it's not just the calories you consume that make the difference in your ability to drop unwanted pounds. It's the inflammation that some foods cause because when a body is in a state of chronic inflammation (which you may not even realize), it affects your metabolism.

The good news is that there are certain foods and habits that can reduce inflammation in the body, which makes whatever fat-reducing, the fitness-enhancing program you do even more effective!

The Link Between Inflammation and Weight Loss

Leptin is a hormone that regulates your body's fat retention by controlling your appetite and metabolism. But chronic inflammation impairs the brain's ability to receive leptin's instructions to your body to suppress the appetite and metabolize foods effectively. Moreover, fat cells are capable of creating chemical signals that lead to chronic inflammation, which they do when you eat too many calories and sugar.

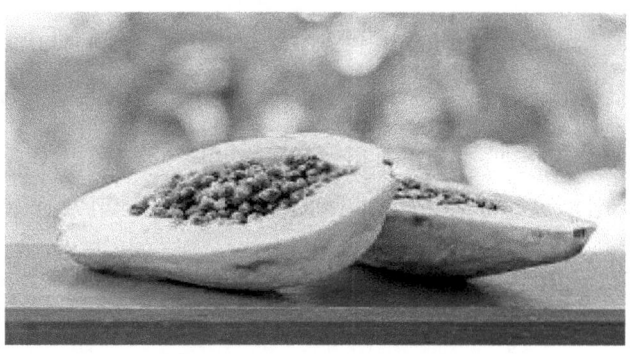

How to lose weight by eating anti-inflammatory foods

Eating foods to reduce inflammation will not only

improve your overall health, but it also improves your body's responsiveness to leptin, making it far easier to take off unwanted pounds without doing anything extreme.

The first step is to remove foods from your diet that cause inflammation in the first place. These are sugary foods, processed foods, and carbs like bread. Incidentally, some people are very sensitive to carbs and have insulin problems, and others are not, so for many, eating carbs is not a huge worry. Nevertheless, if you want to reduce inflammation for weight loss, it's a good idea to limit foods like bread and pasta, and choose whole grains like brown rice or quinoa instead (as I explain below). As a general rule, if food is not in its natural state, then don't eat it. In other words, you should eat food that is basically in the same state it was in when it was in nature, minus the cooking! So say goodbye to biscuits, crackers, and most packaged foods.

Steps To Reduce inflammation in Your Life

Consider the 'Mediterranean Diet' - This diet is

naturally anti-inflammatory and prioritizes fresh fruits, vegetables, and healthy fats. It recommends consuming fatty seafood, eating moderate amounts of nuts; a little red meat; and drinking moderate amounts of red wine.

Include sources of omega-3 fatty acids Omega-3s - inhibit an enzyme that produces prostaglandins, which trigger inflammation. They are found in walnuts, avocados, olive oil, and cold water fish like tuna, salmon, and mackerel.

- Choose more of these veggies and fruits- Broccoli, brussels sprout, kale, cauliflower and other green leafy veggies as they contain sulforaphane, which blocks enzymes linked to inflammation. As for anti-inflammatory fruit, choose papaya, pineapple, cherries, watermelon.

- Choose whole grains if you eat carbs - This means eating brown rice, quinoa, or bulgur wheat rather than white rice or potatoes. The fibre in whole grains reduces the body's inflammatory processes during metabolism.

- Eat specific spices and herbs: You can add them to your cooking, or garnish meals with them - or even combine them to make a tea. Ginger, rosemary, turmeric, oregano, cayenne, cloves, cinnamon, and lemongrass are considered anti-inflammatory.

- Exercise -A recent study has shown that even 20 minutes of exercise a day can lower inflammation in the body.

- Once you've integrated some of these changes in your life, your metabolism can respond, and your ability to lose weight naturally improves. All the best!

Why an Anti-Inflammatory Diet Can Naturally Help You Manage or Lose Weight

Inflammation is known to be the root cause of multiple forms of the disease, ranging from heart disease to diabetes, cancer, arthritis, and many digestive disorders. It's also one of the most overlooked causes of weight problems. Weight loss diets will come and go, and while some may work temporarily to lower the number on the scale, many create larger problems over time due to the fact they rob the body of nutrients and contribute to inflammation. One of these examples is the low-fat craze that took place years ago with fat-free cereals, cookies, chips, peanut butter ... you name it. Then there was the Slim Fast approach, nothing but chemical concoctions dressed up with fancy marketing, and later came diets that involved counting, routine measuring, and other less-than-optimal approaches.

We can all agree that got us nowhere except malnourished, hungry all the time, and likely with more food cravings than when we ever dreamed of. This isn't how nature intended for the body to work. This way of living is not what eating is about, nor is it what our bodies require to be healthy or maintain an optimal weight—which is different for everyone.

Nutritional Balance

When it comes to managing your weight, nutritional balance and consistency are important. Various ups and downs throughout the years aren't healthy for the body, not to mention confusing.Extremely low (or high) calorie diets are naturally inflammatory to the body; they put a strain on the cells and major organs.They can also interfere with other processes of the body ranging from heart, digestive, blood, and other functions.These problems alone also lead to inflammation, repeating a vicious cycle.

The best way to end the cycle and achieve health is to eat a diet that both treats and prevents inflammation, an in return, disease. Most people don't consider the way this leads to a healthy weight, but it's the easiest and most powerful way to lose weight and manage a healthy weight for a longer period. The simple answer?Eat an anti-inflammatory diet based off of whole, plant-based foods.

- Heart Health - A healthy weight is hard to achieve if your heart isn't in good health because the heart controls multiple aspects of metabolism and energy levels. A healthy heart can also help prevent inflammation that leads to diabetes and chronic inflammation that leads to heart disease. It's also more important to focus on heart-healthy foods rather than just how many calories a food has. Some of the best heart-healthy foods include vegetables, nuts, seeds, greens, fruits, beans, legumes, and low-glycemic grains. These are simple enough to get in a plant-based diet, but should also be considered for heart health on any type of diet.

- Anti-inflammatory foods support healthy blood flow, help keep the arteries clear, and help manage hormone levels in our blood, along with blood viscosity necessary to prevent heart disease and diabetes further.

- Food Cravings - Food cravings can also be caused by inflammation, namely sugar, red meat, fried foods, junk foods, and refined grains. These foods don't just make us gain weight, but they stimulate our appetites more because they don't satisfy us nutritionally. The body confuses this unmet need with heightened hunger. Many (refined, processed, and fried foods) also contain ingredients that can trigger a false increased appetite, such as excess salt, sugar, MSG, and various chemicals. Not to mention, many of these foods have been linked to diabetes that leads to problems managing one's weight. Anti-inflammatory foods, on the other hand, such as greens, vegetables, fruits, nuts and seeds, are extremely alkaline and are some of the most nutrient-dense foods we have available to us.

- When the body eats these foods and receives raw nutrients, it is immediately satisfied, given the right fuel to maintain healthy organ function, and no longer suffers because it's not being deprived of real food.

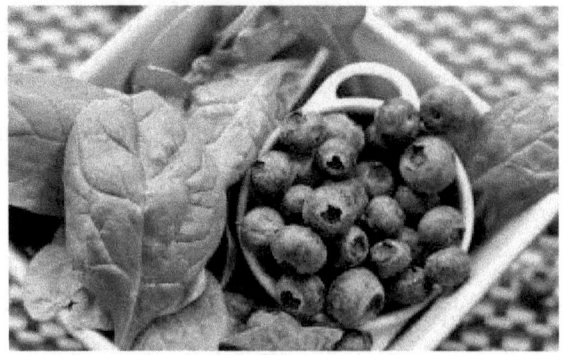

- Blood Sugar - Blood sugar levels are also supported naturally through anti-inflammatory foods; some of the best are natural sources of protein such as hemp seeds, pumpkin seeds, almonds, chia, flax, broccoli, spinach, kale, lentils, and chickpeas. Most all nuts, seeds, greens, vegetables, beans, and legumes support blood sugar levels. While fruits and grains may (and sometimes should) be limited to support blood sugar levels, most people who embrace moderate servings of them still experience better blood sugar levels than excessive amounts of insulin-raising animal proteins.

- When our blood sugar is supported, the

hormones insulin and cortisol are managed much better; this is key to achieving and maintaining a healthy weight, heart and mood health.

- It Maximizes the Good Stuff - More importantly, an anti-inflammatory diet maximizes beneficial foods and reduces the attention to poorer choices. You needn't spend money on diet products, fancy foods, or freezable, low-calorie meals. You also don't need to skip a meal just so you can eat a fast food meal later without feeling guilty, or even exercise all your calories away. An anti-inflammatory diet puts more attention on healthy foods and includes no restriction on calories—when the body receives nutrients it needs; it will naturally let you know when you're full. An anti-inflammatory diet also includes plenty of herbs, spices, and teas which are potent in their abilities to not only reduce inflammation but also satisfy the appetite and palate naturally. Some can even reduce inflammation themselves, such as turmeric, green tea, cilantro, and parsley.

- It's Balanced - An anti-inflammatory diet is also balanced. It does not emphasize one food group over another but embraces healthy fats, anti-inflammatory proteins, and low-glycemic, fibre rich choices of natural carbohydrates. Different amounts of these foods will work differently for each, but a balance much easier to reach when you focus on eating a variety of anti-inflammatory plant-based choices and working them in throughout the day.

These foods are full of vitamins, minerals, amino acids, enzymes, and some even have probiotics and immune-boosting properties which are also linked to weight management and a healthy body.

It should also be noted that an anti-inflammatory diet naturally enables us to move more and be more active. We all sit so much when working or while watching entertainment, surfing the web, dining in restaurants (versus cooking more at home), in our cars, etc. But our bodies can become inflammatory by too much sitting, as they need movement and regular activity for proper lymphatic flow. An inflammatory diet only feeds this as it robs your energy, weakens your joints and immune system, and makes you feel too tired to want to do anything else. To break the cycle, focus on eating anti-inflammatory foods first, and then start moving more. You'll see how much differently healthy foods make you feel, and your body won't be able to stand sitting so much for very long! Walking, yoga and low-intensity exercises also improve lymphatic flow that reduces inflammation in return.

Chapter:-4

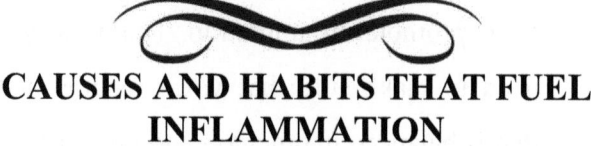

CAUSES AND HABITS THAT FUEL INFLAMMATION

What Causes Inflammation? 4 Factors to Consider

Inflammation is not evil. It is the result of the body's response to infections and other foreign invaders. The problem starts when there is too much of this going on in the body. What causes inflammation? Here are some examples that you might not even realize.

- Diet - If you frequently experience different forms of inflammation, the first thing you should check is your diet. Here's a look at what causes inflammation through the foods you consume.

- Polyunsaturated vegetable oils - corn, peanut, soy, and sunflower are some examples of oil that are high in their content of linoleic acid, an omega-6 fatty acid. Unlike omega-3 fatty acids that relieve inflammation, omega-6 fatty acids promote inflammation. This is why you need to make sure that you consume a diet that is balanced in omega-3 and omega-6.

- Refined carbohydrates - the inflammation reaction to carbohydrates differs from person to person. Based on research, however, the more the carbohydrate has undergone processing, the faster it is converted to blood glucose and the higher the glycemic index. When the glycemic index is high, the more insulin is released, which is one of the causes of inflammation.

- Red meat - studies have shown that a molecule (the sugar found in non-human mammals) become absorbed in the tissues of persons consuming certain types of red meats. Subsequent tests have shown that the presence of this type of sugar (that human are unable to produce genetically) in the body can trigger an immune system response that is one of the inflammation causes.

Then there are other factors that cause inflammation:

- Stress - Whenever we undergo trying situations, the body releases the stress hormone cortisol through the adrenal glands.

- Cortisol raises blood pressure and blood sugar levels to help you survive the short bouts of stress. However, its long-term effect is bad.

- So, what causes inflammation when a person is stressed? Although cortisol is an anti-inflammatory hormone, all it does is suppress parts of the immune system. This means that while cortisol is doing its job, the immune system is unable to fight new infections that affect the body, which can lead to more health problems.

- Environment - Air fresheners, adhesives, glue, cleaning products, pollution, pesticides - these are just some of the chemicals we expose ourselves to every day. Whether you are in your workplace, on the streets, and even inside your house, there is the possibility that you and your family are not safe from these irritants.

- The effect on the immune system differs from person to person because of the varying levels of immunity that everyone has. Nevertheless, constant exposure to these chemicals can someday trigger an immune system response that can lead to inflammation.

- Menopause - There are many changes in a woman's body during menopause. One of which is the loss of hormones that were present in the early stages of life.

Studies have shown that the loss of hormones may lead to chronic inflammation.

In turn, chronic inflammation has been associated with osteoporosis, cancer, heart disease, and other autoimmune diseases.Furthermore, chronic inflammation causes the body to attack itself. This means that the immune system, which responds to infections, keeps attacking even when there is no longer any danger.

What causes inflammation? This question was answered by the examples stated. Your body's response to the factors above may be different. This is why it is important for you to be attuned to your body so you will know how to better take care of it.

Daily Habits That Can Age You

The anti-aging industry is a multi-billion dollar industry (and growing), proving that the quest for the elusive fountain of youth continues. Millions of people worldwide routinely apply topical anti-aging creams, undergo speciality treatments and try various vitamins and diets in the hopes of finding the cure to aging. According to MedHelp.org, as many of us practice habits of staying young and healthy, some of our daily habits are actually speeding the aging clock and making us unhealthy. The following are some of the harmful habits that may be having a negative effect on your skin and health.

Skimping on sleep

It's normal to suffer from periodic lack of sleep, but routinely getting to bed late and waking up groggy can take its toll on your skin. Sleeping is your body's time to rest and repair cell damage. People who don't get a good night's sleep show signs of premature skin aging, where their skin appears dull and sallow. Chronic lack of sleep has also been linked to obesity, diabetes, heart disease, poor immune function and ultimately, a shorter life expectancy.

Sugar Shock

Too much sugar can cause premature wrinkles and sagging skin. According to Huffingtonpost.com, when there is excess sugar in the body, it attaches itself to collagen, causing the skin to look stiff and lose its flexibility. Losing this elasticity will give the skin deep wrinkles and make it look weathered. A diet high in simple sugars - cakes, soda, and candy - causes glucose spikes that cause inflammation, which can also lead to premature aging.

Forgetting your sunglasses

The original purpose of sunglasses (before they became a must-have accessory) was to shield and protect the eyes against the sun. Routinely squinting to avoid the brightness of the sun can cause fine lines and wrinkles to form around your eyes. More importantly, exposing your eyes to UV rays can lead to cataracts, macular degeneration, and skin cancers which can occur inside the eye and on the eyelid.

No downtime

Having a demanding schedule and being chronically under stress can have a negative impact on your mind and body health. It's important to take time regularly to relax your mind and body. Practising relaxation techniques such as deep breathing, guided imagery and yoga can help prevent heart disease, digestive issues, obesity, and a weakened immune system.

Excessive drinking

Studies repeatedly show the benefits red wine has on preventing heart disease and reducing bad cholesterol. While one glass of wine can benefit your health, drinking excessively can harm your liver, raise blood pressure, cause certain cancers and make your skin look dehydrated and tired.

You've eliminated all fat from your diet

Eliminating certain fats - saturated and trans fats - from your diet is a wise heart-healthy move. But not all fats are bad. Omega-3 fatty acids, like those found in fish, nuts, and olive oil, are the ultimate anti-aging fat, essential for protecting your cardiovascular health, brain, bones, joints, skin, and more. According to Prevention.com, monounsaturated fat can lower bad LDL cholesterol, raise cardio-protective HDL cholesterol, and decrease your risk of atherosclerosis.

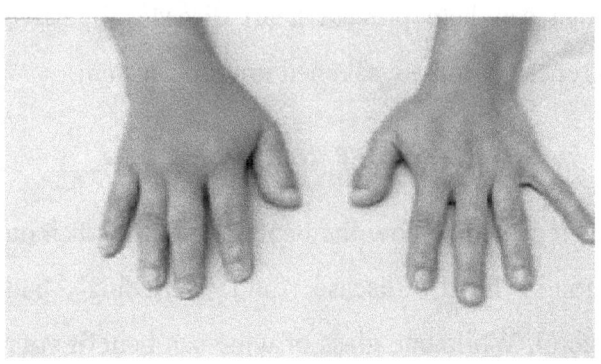

Foods to Avoid for Preventing Inflammation

As the old saying goes, "the bigger they are, the harder the fall." Same goes with inflammation and other dietary problems. But all hope is never lost. Inflammation, acidity and other such problems are common today thanks to all the junk food that we eat and also due to the sedentary lifestyle and lack of physical exercise. Moreover, the amount of mental you face to keep up in the rat race is also one of the major reasons. I simply cannot stress enough on the virtues of having a balanced diet and avoiding all of the above problems but for now let us concentrate more on the cures and prevention measures for inflammation and even before that, the causes of inflammation.

The main ingredients causing inflammation are proteins called cytokines.And it is your diet that plays an important role in suppressing or activating these proteins. These proteins are also toxic to the body and pollute the internal passages of your body and in particular, the intestines and lead to inflammation.

You need to understand that whatever you consume

is going to have some effect, good or bad on your body and based on that you decide what foods to consume and what is best avoided. Remember, there is no neutrality as far as food is concerned. They are either good for you or bad. But everything consumed in moderation is good. And here is a basic list of foods that are notorious for producing more of cytokines, the inflammatory protein.

- Meats, especially Red Meat except for fish that are oily - Only fish that are oily do not cause inflammation. Moreover, red meat is harmful in many other ways too if over-consumed. Many people who want to lose weight and opt for diets that are low on carbohydrates often tend to consume a lot of red meat as it I known to be low on fattening fats, carbohydrates and cholesterol. The ideal quantity of red meat for those who wish to prevent inflammation should be around four ounces per week. To compensate for the protein intake, opt for foods that are rich on vegetarian proteins.

- Egg Yolks - Egg yolks are known to be high on acid, viz.; arachidonic acid that causes inflammation. This is also the same substance that makes all forms of meat cause inflammation. It is ideally advised by doctors that one consumes only the white part of eggs.

- Dairy Products - Dairy products including milk are also high on the same arachidonic acid, and it is often observed that in countries like Sweden, the United Kingdom and even Canada where dairy products are consumed in substantially high quantities are most susceptible to inflammation and even osteoporosis; a disease which leads to the weakening and even breaking of bones.

- Milk often referred to as the complete food has also many vices such as aggravating asthma, and it is known to even contain some addictive endorphins and even certain narcotic substances.

- Corn & Corn Oils and Syrups - Corn is

known to contain fructose besides cytokines. It is the combination of these two that is highly addictive and is known to be present even in cigarettes. Manufacturers of cigarettes have been using corn syrup since as early as World War I, not for the good taste that it has but for the fact that it is addictive.

- Sugar - Sugar in all its forms is known to cause inflammation on prolonged consumption and overdose. Moreover, it also causes obesity & weight gain. Studies and surveys show that an average America consumes as much as a hundred and fifty-three pounds of refined sugar that is known to be highly difficult to digest and this prevents the body from absorbing the nutrients in it such as minerals and vitamins. Moreover, sugar is even dehydrating.

Six Common Foods That Contribute to Inflammation

Many of the foods common to American diets today

are now known to contribute to a chain of events known as the Inflammation Cascade. Experts say that reducing or eliminating these foods from your diet can significantly reduce pain and inflammation in muscles and joints.

- Cereals and Grains - Archeologists have found evidence that soon after farming and consuming larger amounts of these foods that signs of health problems and afflictions began to emerge and become more prevalent in human society.

- Cereals and grains, mostly in the form of bread and pasta, make up a large part of today's average American diet. What most people don't realize is that all grains are highly acidic, and also contain gluten, a common allergen. Most bread and pasta are made with highly processed and bleached flours, which increase their acidity as well. Starches in these foods are broken down by your body into sugars, which are then stored as fat.

- Even so-called "whole grain" products often start with the same processed, bleached-out flour, and have their "whole grains" added later. Read the label carefully to make sure it docsn't contain "refined flour" or "refined wheat flour" to know that it is made from whole grains.

- Oils - Polyunsaturated oils, like safflower, sunflower, corn, peanut, and soy, are high in omega-6 fatty acids that your body converts to arachidonic acid. Arachidonic acid has a pro-inflammatory influence on the body. These oils also contain almost no omega-3 fatty acids, found in flaxseed and olive oils, which are known to soothe inflammation. Trans-fats, hydrogenated, and partially hydrogenated oils should be avoided as well since these create free-radicals which are foods that cause inflammation.

- Refined Sugars - High levels of insulin in the body trigger our immune systems, as well as activating enzymes that raise levels of arachidonic acids in our blood, leading to inflammation. Processed sugars, such as high-fructose corn syrup, and foods that are known to have high glycemic indexes cause a spike in the body's insulin levels. The Glycemic Index (GI) is a system for rating carbohydrates, or saccharides, based on their immediate effect on the blood glucose level.

- Processed Meats - Highly processed meats, such as lunch meats, sausages, or hot dogs, contain large amounts of nitrites. Nitrites have long been associated with increased inflammation and chronic disease. Often people are born or develop allergies to nitrites without knowing it, and only through a doctors test do they find out they are allergic to certain foods containing nitrites. A simple adjustment to their diet will eliminate many of the reactions they become afflicted with from consuming such foods as processed meats or peanut butter, or bananas.

- Saturated Fats - Saturated fats are found in

red meat, dairy, and eggs. While these foods are an important source of minerals and vitamins, they also contain arachidonic acid. Do not break egg yolks before cooking. When the yolk of an egg, high in saturated fats, is mixed with the white, while still raw, arachidonic acid is formed. Some arachidonic acid in your diet is necessary for proper health, but too much is associated with increased inflammation. Pick lean cuts of red meat to cut down on the number of saturated fats, or stick to poultry, venison, or fish.

- Nightshade Fruits and Vegetables - Although there hasn't been any formal research, it has long been believed that members of the nightshade family of plants, such as tomatoes, potatoes and eggplant, can make inflammation in muscles and joints worse. These vegetables contain a chemical called solanine which can trigger pain and inflammation in some people.

- Allergies over time Note that people develop

allergies over time to some foods and drinks. It stands to reason too, then, that over time you should see a marked improvement in how you feel when you know which foods cause inflammation, and which foods reduce inflammation that you adopt a diet that can relieve pain or perhaps prevent it in the first place.

- So, with all the foods to avoid for inflammation, and all the foods causing inflammation, what can you do?Bodybuilders have long known the value of eating with as much variety as possible to receive as many nutrients from as many different foods as possible.

- With today's vast and ample supplies of conventional supermarkets, as well as the many Asian and Indian markets, it is conceivable that virtually every nutrient and flavor can be enjoyed. Meal planning plus diets rich in nutrients as well as flavours enhanced with spices and herbs from different parts of the world can also be exciting as well as palatable.

Foods that Cause Inflammation

There are foods that you consume every day that give to inflammation. It may not seem important, until the day you come down with a symptom like; arthritis, cancer, or diabetes. These three diseases deal with inflammation, and it is very important to learn about the foods you put in your mouth every day, to help control it.

What are some of the foods that cause inflammation? How many of you get up in the morning and eat these for breakfast, every day?

Bacon

Eggs

Coffee

Dairy products

Many common foods in the Standard North American Diet can cause or exacerbate inflammation in the body.

11 Foods that cause inflammation:

- A processed, package, or prepared foods: Yes, fast foods is at the top of the list of inflammatory foods thanks to the harmful oils, sugar and artificial sweeteners, food additives, and a whole host of nasty ingredients.

- Hydrogenated and trans fats: These are found in margarine, shortening, lard and products made with them. That includes baked goods, cookies, pies, buns. Of course, there are healthier alternatives to these baked goods, but most grocery stores and bakeries are using these harmful ingredients.

- Meat: (Not wild caught fish) A plant-based diet tends much lower in inflammatory substances, but meat and poultry tend to cause inflammation so make them the background of your meals, not the main dish.

- White sugar and sweets: This includes soft drinks and sweetened juices. Research shows that sugar is the most addictive substance you can use, it's also highly inflammatory. No, you do not need to drop sugar and sweets altogether simply cut your consumption and choose fruit as your "go to" food when you're craving something sweet.

- Synthetic sweeteners: Let's list a few you will find on the store shelf today in your local supermarket; NutraSweet, Splenda, saccharin, aspartame, Amino Sweet, etc. Research links these substances to many serious health conditions. You should seriously try your best to avoid these.

- Iodized Salt: (Use Celtic sea salt instead). Not harmful on its own but sodium is naturally found along with other valuable minerals like potassium, calcium, and magnesium. Choose unrefined salt which naturally has many minerals, not just sodium.

- Food additives: colors; flavor enhancers, stabilizers, and perversities. Some of the main ones include sulfites, benzoate, and colors named FD&C #"X." Unfortunately, many foods consumed by children have these harmful, toxic ingredients.

- Dairy products: (Yogurt, ice cream, cottage cheese, butter, cheese, etc.) The reasons dairy products are inflammatory are too lengthy to list here, but today's dairy products contain hormones, antibiotics, and other harmful ingredients so avoid them as much as possible.

- Wheat products: Wheat is highly acid-forming and inflammatory in the body. Worse, most wheat available now is genetically modified (GM). Many serious health conditions are pointing to GM wheat consumption.

- Other gluten-containing grains: Gluten is found in most grains and is highly inflammatory. Choose grains or seeds like buckwheat, guinea, or millet for your backing.

- Alcohol: High is sugar and a burden to the liver, alcohol makes the top of the inflammatory foods list. It is best eliminated or used in moderation.

Learning to curb our appetite from the foods that cause inflammation in your everyday life can lessen the risk of heart attack and stroke in our society today.

CHAPTER:-5

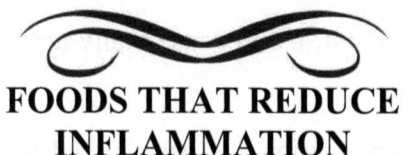

FOODS THAT REDUCE INFLAMMATION

6 Powerful Super-foods That Fight Inflammation

Chronic inflammation seems to be one of the most talked about topics these days. Recently there has been more of a focus on long term inflammation in the body and how it affects us.

Inflammation on its own is not a bad thing, as it is the body's natural response to outside threats, like infections or toxic chemicals.Inflammation also can kick up during stressful situations. Inflammation helps your body repair a wound or fight off an illness. A fever is one example of an inflammation response by your body, or a sore throat and swollen glands. This means your body is sending white blood cells to the area to fight off infection.

However, inflammation should be short-lived, once

the infection is gone the inflammation should subside. When inflammation persists even when there isn't a need for it, it can cause many negative effects on the body.

Chronic inflammation has been linked to damage in the joints (such as from rheumatoid arthritis). Inflammation has also been found to cause heart damage, as fatty plaques within your blood vessels grow larger as white blood cells collect.

These eventually form blood clots, which can block the flow of blood to your heart, leading to a heart attack.

Controlled, temporary inflammation = good. Uncontrolled, chronic inflammation = very bad for your health.

Before we get into the six foods that are best at curbing inflammation, here are some general pointers to improve your diet.

The number one tip I can give you is to stop eating the overly processed foods that are prevalent in many Western diets.

Make sure to stay far away from sugar and grains as

well; it Is vitally important that you limit them in your diet for overall health.

Without further ado, here are six foods that do wonders to help control chronic inflammation.

- Green Leafy Vegetables - One of the top items for a good diet is green leafy vegetables. These unassuming green leaves are high in antioxidants, as well as Vitamin A, C, K.

- Additionally, they are high in flavonoids, which have an anti-inflammatory effect. Some great examples of leafy green vegetables are swiss chard, spinach, kale, bok choy and cabbage.

- One idea is to make a green smoothie to easily and deliciously get your fill of leafy greens! Add your favorite greens, frozen fruit, yoghurt and water in a blender and blend for a delicious, ridiculously healthy treat!

- Celery - In recent studies, celery was found to have both antioxidant and anti-inflammatory abilities that can improve your blood pressure and cholesterol levels.

- Celery is also an excellent source of potassium, which works hand in hand with sodium to bring in nutrients and also flush out the toxins from cells.

- Blueberries - One especially strong antioxidant is known as quercetin, it is effective at fighting inflammation and even cancer. Quercetin is found in citrus, olive oil and dark-colored berries, like blueberries.

- One study found that consuming blueberries slowed cognitive decline and improved memory and motor function. That's incredible for such a small fruit! Give blueberries a try in your green smoothie for a massive antioxidant boost!

- Pineapple - Pineapple is high in a digestive enzyme known as bromelain, which is a known anti-inflammatory and can even optimize your immune system.

- Pineapple is also high in Vitamin C, vitamin B1 and potassium.

- It can even help to heal your heart, by stopping blood platelets from sticking together, the cause of blood clots in your heart.

- Beets - Did you know that a deep color in a fruit or vegetable is one indicator of a high level of antioxidants? Once you understand that, you can see how beets are slammed packed with high impact antioxidants! The antioxidant betalain gives beets their classic color and cell repairing ability.

- Beets are also high in magnesium, and magnesium deficiency has been linked to high levels of inflammation within the body.

- Coconut Oil - The lipids (fatty acids) in coconut oil are strong anti-inflammatory compounds that lower inflammation within the body. In an Indian study, the high levels of antioxidants in virgin coconut oil reduced inflammation and worked to help heal arthritis better than many leading medications.

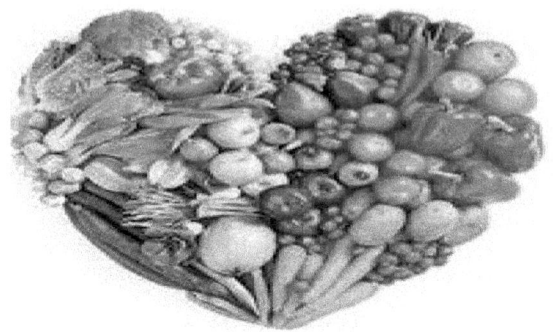

Well, there you have it, six powerful foods that are high in antioxidants and are capable of drastically reducing inflammation within the body.

Remember, first it is vitally important that you eliminate processed foods within your diet, as well as foods high in sugar or grains.

Then you should work on incorporating these healthy foods into your diet, as well as other powerful foods.

I hope this guide helped you to improve your diet and health by lowering inflammation within your body.

One area when it came to optimizing the diet that I had real trouble with was getting the right serving size of these powerful foods. It can be tough finding out the right amount you should be eating every day to fully benefit from the antioxidant effects of these foods.

7 Foods That Reduce Inflammation Naturally

Do you or someone you love suffer from inflammation and the pain that comes with it? If so, I'm happy to share with you a little of what I have learned through my journey to healing my inflammation. I will share with you seven foods that reduce inflammation naturally.

In my early 20's, I dealt with daily pain from inflammation in several areas of my body. So I know how painful and debilitating inflammation can be. When I could take the pain any longer, I decided to take matters into my own hands, and find out how to get rid of my inflammation for good and in a natural way. Before I share some of the secrets I have found, it is important to know what inflammation is. So, what is inflammation?

Inflammation is part of the biological response of

vascular tissues to harmful stimuli. These stimuli could be damaged cells, pathogens, or irritants. Inflammation is a protective attempt by your body to remove the detrimental stimuli and to start the healing process. Infections and wounds would never heal without inflammation. Symptoms of inflammation can include swelling, pain, redness, and restriction in movement.

Inflammation can be acute or chronic.Chronic inflammation is prolonged inflammation. It leads to a progressive shift in the type of cells existing at the site of inflammation and is characterized by concurring destruction and healing of the tissue from the inflammatory process. It can cause a load of diseases, such as arthritis, rheumatoid arthritis, periodontitis, hay fever, cancer, inflammatory bowel diseases, hypersensitivities, diabetes, stroke, heart disease, acne, celiac disease, autoimmune diseases, asthma, etc. So for that reason, the body closely regulates inflammation.

It is important to reduce inflammation not just because of the pain that it causes you, but also because chronic inflammation is very detrimental to the body. Unlike acute inflammation, where the immune system responds to injury or infection by activating inflammatory chemicals that fight abnormal substances, chronic inflammation isn't beneficial for the body.

The foods you choose to eat can help reduce and prevent inflammation. Foods reduce inflammation naturally, so if you want to get rid of your inflammation naturally, then read on! Below I will share with you seven foods that reduce inflammation naturally. These foods are called anti-inflammatory foods.

- Berries - Goji berries are one of the first foods I choose to eat to rid myself of my horrible inflammation pain, and I noticed a difference within weeks. Goji berries are very high in antioxidants, so they are a great anti-inflammatory along with other wonderful qualities. Blueberries are full of antioxidants and high in phytonutrients. Phytonutrients give anti-inflammatory protection against many diseases. Other types of berries such as raspberries, blackberries, strawberries and cranberries are also high in antioxidants.

- Papaya - Papain is a protein-digesting enzyme found in papaya. Papain, along with other nutrients such as vitamin E and C, helps to reduce inflammation and improves digestion. If you are interested in foods that reduce inflammation, and you are a tropical fruit fan, then this is a perfect food for you to eat.

- Pineapple - Pineapple contains bromelain, an enzyme that aids in the healing of indigestion, sports injury, trauma and other kinds of swelling and inflammation. Extracts of bromelain are used in various natural anti-inflammatory supplements for arthritis.

- Spices - Turmeric is a spice with high anti-inflammatory qualities. Add a teaspoon to your diet each day. Some ways to include turmeric into your diet would be to add it to soups, sprinkling it on scrambled eggs, mixing it into sauces, or salad dressings.

Ginger is a relative of turmeric that is also revered internationally for its anti-inflammatory qualities. If you want to reduce inflammation naturally, then try incorporating these spices in your next meals.

- Kelp - Kelp contains fucoidan, a kind of carbohydrate that is anti-inflammatory, and anti-oxidative. Kombu, arame, and wakame are a few types of kelp that can be bought at the grocery store. Kelp has a high fibre content, so it also helps to make you feel full and promotes weight loss. Get organic kelp from unpolluted waters.

- Spinach - Spinach is a dark green leafy vegetable that is a high source of anti-inflammatory and anti-oxidative flavonoids and carotenoids. It contains vitamin A, B, B, C, E, K, iron, magnesium, potassium, calcium, and folate. Make sure to buy organic spinach. Non-organic spinach is sprayed with pesticides, and you don't want to be putting more toxins into your body, because that will increase your inflammation. Vegetables, especially dark leafy vegetables are great for decreases inflammation. Choose dark green or brightly colored vegetables.

- Broccoli - Broccoli contains anti-inflammatory phytonutrients that help the body to get rid of carcinogenic compounds. It is also a highly nutritious vegetable. Cauliflower is a relative of broccoli, which contains similar components that aid the body's detoxification.

- I hope you have found this list of foods that reduce inflammation helpful. Start eating some of these foods, and see what happens. If you already eat some of them, try eating more. The more you eat of these foods, the more you should see a reduction in your inflammation and the pain that goes with it. Here's to a new you... inflammation and pain-free!

6 Healthy Eating Habits to Stop Chronic Inflammation

Did you know that inflammation is a silent killer? Did you know that you can reduce chronic inflammation through diet?

Below are 6 Healthy Eating Habits to STOP Chronic Inflammation:

- Eat 5 Servings of Vegetables: It's important to eat a variety of veggies. Vegetables are high in vitamins, minerals and fiber. Include a variety of "colors" each day such as sweet potatoes, spinach and squash. A serving is ½ cup cooked or 1 cup of raw. Mix it up and eat both raw and cooked. A salad is an easy way to get multiple veggies in one meal.

- Eat 3 to 4 Servings of Fruit: If you're trying to lose weight eat the lesser and for optimal health eat 4 servings per day. Again, eat a variety of colors and pick fresh fruit over dried or juice as much as possible. Berries are a great choice as they are low glycemic and high in fiber, eat them daily. An apple a day keeps the doctor away! A serving is ½ cup or a small piece. It is best to eat fruit with protein, have some nuts or yoghurt with your fruit.

- Eat Lean Protein: It is best to eat white lean protein like fish, chicken and turkey most of the time. If you happen to like red meat it's OK to eat it once or twice a week, make sure it's lean. Other sources of protein are nuts and soy. Nuts are a great way to add protein, fiber and healthy fat to your diet. Just make sure you don't eat too many - about ¼ cup is a serving. Soy can be a great alternative to meat. Try tofu dishes and veggie burgers for a change twice a week.

- Eat 3 Servings of Carbs: Make sure the grains you're consuming are Whole Grains only. A good rule of thumb is to make sure the carbs you're eating also contain at least 2-5 grams of fiber. This slows the conversion of starch to sugar. Whole grain bread, whole wheat pasta, oatmeal and brown rice are good choices. Try rye cereal for something different. Add soy milk, berries and top with nuts for a healthy balanced breakfast.

- Fats: Don't eliminate fat from your diet. It is very important to have them with every meal. The healthy fats are olive oil, coconut oil, nuts and avocado. Stay away from trans fats because they raise bad cholesterol and lower good cholesterol. This combination is what causes inflammation and has a negative effect on your health. Become a smart reader of labels. Steer away from hydrogenated and partially hydrogenated fats.

- Daily Supplements: Vitamins, minerals, antioxidants and fish oil taken daily can lower levels of inflammation in the body. Be sure to take multivitamins and multi-minerals to get all of the essential nutrients needed. Remember vitamins need minerals for proper absorption and vice versa, so be sure to take both twice daily. When purchasing supplements look for natural and pharmaceutical grade to ensure you're getting what is stated on the label and it's pure and bioavailable to the body.

If you incorporate these recommendations to your diet on a regular basis you will be on your way to optimal health. One last thing...exercise daily because exercise also reduces inflammation.

3 Top Keys to Prevent Inflammation

Inflammation can be a two-edged sword. There are two types of inflammation: acute and chronic (or silent). Acute inflammation gets your attention right away such as with an athletic injury - it hurts. But silent inflammation is a result of our immune system that goes out of control. It is much like putting gasoline on an already burning fire. It is insidious because it goes on 24 hours a day. You cannot feel silent inflammation until the cumulative damage begins to talk to us, if you will, in the form of diabetes, arthritis, weight gain, heart disease, Alzheimer's Disease, cancer, faster aging, symptoms and much more.

What is the pay-off for reducing or preventing inflammation? You will think with clarity, have more energy, and prevent illness, disease and symptoms and as a bonus? You will look younger, healthier and more vibrant.

Cooling the heat of inflammation starts with these three tips:

Avoid Foods That Trigger Inflammation

The first step in cooling the heat of inflammation on a cellular level is to pay attention to your diet.

- Avoid the following foods:

- Poor fats, Polyunsaturated vegetable oils such as cottonseed, safflower, corn, sunflower oils and commercially prepared peanut butter.

- Partially Hydrogenated Vegetable Oil(trans fat) found in many packaged and processed foods, deep fried foods, fast foods, commercial baked goods and those prepared with partially hydrogenated oil, margarine and vegetable shortening.

- Sugars of all varieties including fruit juice.

- Refined carbohydrates such as white flour

products, white rice, and white bread, desserts and processed foods.

Exercise is Powerful.

Exercising only occasionally can trigger inflammation but a consistent program most days of the week is a powerful tool in preventing and reducing the inflammatory response. There is a strong correlation between exercise and reducing whole body inflammation. The use of exercise is key in creating optimal health and longevity.

For example, exercise can prevent heart disease which is now thought to be a result of poor lifestyle choices and these choices can lead to not only heart disease but other inflammatory conditions as well. Many studies have found that exercise reduces C-reactive protein and other inflammatory compounds. Exercise also raises your good cholesterol (HDL), helps with anxiety and depression, builds strong muscle and bone which is important to optimal health and has a tremendous impact on our emotional health as well.

Supplements Are Necessary

If you want to fight disease and achieve maximum life span, you can't do it with diet alone. You need the extra nutritional boost that only supplements can provide.

We are a nation plagued with nutrient deficiencies for a variety of reasons. Poor diet stands at the forefront, but stress, allergies, pollution, smoking, and allergies, all contribute to a lack of optimal health. Depending on how long our food is stored, the number of pesticides used, whether organic or conventional and often our conventional food is grown in nutrient-depleted soil. And lastly, some individuals require more of certain nutrients than others.

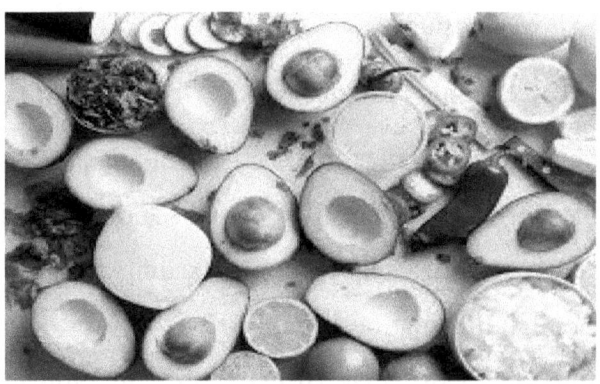

We need to ensure that our antioxidant and nutrient intake is high to help keep inflammation in check. In doing so, you will not only protect against deficiency but create optimal health as well.

The following supplements are key to preventing or reducing inflammation:

- Multiple Vitamin/Mineral
- B-Complex Vitamin (100 mg)
- Vitamin C (2,000 mg)
- Resveratrol (150 mg)
- Alpha Lipoic Acid (50 mg)
- CoQ10 (100 mg)
- Calcium/Magnesium (1,000 Calcium/600 Magnesium)
- Curcumin (150 mg)

Eating foods high in antioxidants, avoiding processed foods, drinking plenty of water and exercising regularly will all help with the healing process by reducing inflammation in your body.

Avoiding foods that trigger the inflammatory

response, exercising and adding supplements, you will profoundly prevent and reduce inflammation.

Dangers of Microwave Cooking

Yes, there is no doubt that the microwave oven was one of the eighties hottest must-have kitchen appliances. Do you remember how much the first ones cost to own? Look how cheap and common they have become since. Sure heating foods and liquids in seconds, not minutes, has caused most people to abandon any intuitively negative thought they may have had in suspecting radiation cooking to be bad for you. Due to this convenience factor, denying and not acknowledging the danger is normal. But, there are reasons why the sale of these appliances was banned early on in countries like the Soviet Union.

One of the worst outcomes of microwaved food is not so much the radiation factor, as most people feared, but the almost complete (97%) nutrient loss in healthy fresh food like vegetables, for instance, when micro-cooked. There is also the formation of new radiolytic compounds. This chemical structure change in foods and liquids has been the focus of a few studies done to determine what kinds of changes occur in microwaved foods. Rest assured, however, that although the studies have been few, the changes discovered have been significant.

Hans Hartel, a Swiss food scientist, is a man of intense passion, he determined that there is no need to violate the laws of nature by corporate man and his state-supported monopolies in science, technology, or education. Hans was one of the first scientists to form an idea to conduct a qualitative study on the effects of microwaved nutrients had on the blood and physiology of human beings. This small but well-controlled study pointed a very firm finger at a highly degenerative force in microwave ovens and the food produced in them.

Blood samples of the volunteer test subjects were taken before the ingestion of the foods offered. Then, at predetermined intervals after the eating of raw milk and raw vegetables or the same food conventionally cooked, or microwaved.

What was eye-opening, and rather shocking, was that

there were significant changes discovered in the blood samples of the test subjects who had eaten the foods cooked in a microwave oven. These changes included a decrease in all haemoglobin and cholesterol values, especially between the HDL (good cholesterol) and LDL (bad cholesterol) values and ratio.

White blood cells also showed a more distinct short-term decrease after eating microwaved food than opposed to eating food conventionally cooked or raw. Hartel's conclusion was this, due to extensive scientific literature describing the different hazardous effects that microwave radiation has on living systems, it is astonishing what little effort has been made to replace this technology with something more nature-friendly.

From the conclusions of Swiss, Russian, and German scientific studies, here are ten good reasons to ditch your microwave oven for good.

- Continually eating food processed from a microwave oven causes long term - permanent- brain damage by "shorting out"electrical impulses in the brain [depolarizing or de-magnetizing the brain tissue].

- The human body cannot metabolize [break down] the unknown by-products created in microwaved food.

- Male and female hormone production is shut down and altered by continually eating microwaved foods.

- The effects of microwaved food by-products are residual [long term, permanent] within the human body.

- Minerals, vitamins, and other nutrients of all microwaved food are reduced or altered so that the human body gets little or no benefit, or the human body absorbs altered compounds that cannot be broken down.

- The minerals in vegetables are altered into cancerous free radicals when cooked in microwave ovens.

- Microwaved foods cause stomach and

intestinal cancerous growths [tumors]. This may explain the rapidly increasing rate of colon cancer in America.

- The prolonged eating of microwaved foods causes cancerous cells to increase in human blood.

- Continual ingestion of microwaved foods causes immune system deficiencies through lymph gland and blood serum alterations.

- Eating microwaved food causes loss of memory, concentration, emotional instability, and a decrease of intelligence.

CHAPTER:-6

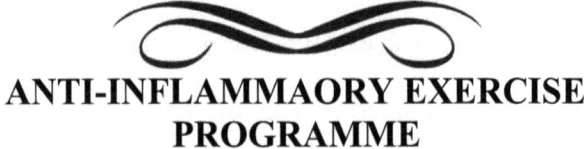

ANTI-INFLAMMAORY EXERCISE PROGRAMME

The Exercise and Body Inflammation Relationship

In the course of fighting inflammation, it is important to make the connection between anti-inflammatory exercise and whole body inflammation. On an Anti-Inflammatory Diet & Exercise Program, you'll exercise at least five days a week, for at least 30 minutes. Start by trying to achieve 50-75% of the maximum heart rate for your age. You may need to do intervals at first to get enough quality exercise. As you get in shape, increase your working heart rate to 70-85% of maximum, with three days of aerobic exercise (walking, running, elliptical) and two days of circuit training: aerobic exercise to warm up and cool down, combined with a resistant, weight-training program designed to work for 8-10 muscle groups. By making the exercise and inflammation connection, this approach has been shown to markedly reduce inflammatory messengers and whole body inflammation.

Exercise to Reduce Whole Body Inflammation

In an anti-inflammation Program, the leading reason to exercise is to reduce whole body inflammation. That's right; there is a strong connection between exercise and whole body inflammation if done the right way. The data on the association between exercise and inflammation is far more positive and conclusive than for exercise and weight loss.

Observational studies reveal that you're 47 per cent less likely to have elevated levels of the inflammatory messenger C-reactive protein (CRP) if you exercise regularly, compared to being sedentary. CRP is a marker of whole body inflammation. Fitness is a separate and independent factor in regulating chronic low-grade inflammation (whole body inflammation). An interventional study conducted by researchers at Louisiana State University demonstrated that aerobic and resistance training very similar to the exercise approach in anti-inflammatory exercise Program reduced CRP levels in both old and young participants by 50 to 60 per cent. These are huge effects on whole body inflammation and are further evidence of the relationship between exercise and inflammation.

Shifting the Fitness Paradigm: Whole Body Inflammation vs Weight Loss

Exercising to Reduce Whole Body Inflammation vs Exercising to Lose Weight

The primary role of exercise in the anti-inflammatory exercise Program is its role in reducing whole body inflammation. It's not that you can't lose weight by exercising. You can. The weight-loss equation boils down to burning more calories than you take in, and exercise is a way to burn calories. But it's a pretty inefficient system, and sets up a lot of people for failure.

Think of it this way: To burn 100 calories, you'd

have to bike at 5 miles per hour for 32 minutes, walk at 3 miles per hour for 23 minutes, swim slowly for 20 minutes, or engage in vigorous aerobic activity for 10 minutes. That's a lot of work! By comparison, it's easy to consume 100 calories; you can do it in the blink of an eye. Just eat one medium-size banana, one medium-to-large apple, or 1 ounce of American cheese. One cup of sweet tea or a cookie, and—calorically speaking—you might as well have skipped your bike ride altogether.

Not to mention that when you exercise a lot, your body compensates with mechanisms to maintain your current weight. For example, it naturally decreases your non-exercise-induced energy expenditure—that is, the calories you burn just engaging in normal activities of daily living, like sitting at your desk.

Exercise and InflammationWhat You'll Need for Your Anti-inflammatory Work Outs

Don't tell the athletic gear companies, but you don't need too many accessories to get a good workout designed to reduce whole body inflammation. You'll need some way to get your heart rate up—whether that's the elliptical machine at the gym or the hill outside your door (both work equally well)—and you'll need some hand weights. The type of mat used for yoga and Pilates can also be helpful if you like a little padding when you stretch. An exercise ball and exercise bands are helpful as well. A heart rate monitor will help you know when you are exercising at your target heart rate.

And while a fancy outfit isn't necessary, we strongly recommend that you invest in good-quality, properly-fitted sneakers.

Weekly Plan Overview – Exercise to Reduce Whole Body Inflammation

FIRST WEEK

SATURDAY - 30 min Light Exercise

SUNDAY - Light Circuit

MONDAY - 30 min Moderate Exercise

TUESDAY – REST

WEDNESDAY - - Moderate Exercise 30 min

THURSDAY - Light Circuit

FRIDAY - REST

SECOND WEEK

SATURDAY - 30 min Light Exercise

SUNDAY - Light Circuit

MONDAY - 30 min Moderate Exercise

TUESDAY - REST

WEDNESDAY - Moderate Exercise 30 min

THURSDAY - Light Circuit

FRIDAY - REST

THIRD WEEK

SATURDAY - 30 min Light Exercise

SUNDAY - Light Circuit

MONDAY - 30 min Moderate Exercise

TUESDAY - REST

WEDNESDAY - 30 min Moderate Exercise

THURSDAY - Light Circuit

FRIDAY - REST

FOURTH WEEK

SATURDAY - 30 min Light Exercise

SUNDAY - Light Circuit

MONDAY - 30 min Moderate Exercise

TUESDAY - REST

WEDNESDAY - 30 min Moderate Exercise

THURSDAY - Light Circuit

FRIDAY - REST

CHAPTER:-7
ANTI-INFLAMMATORY SUPPLEMENTS AND OTHER RELATED ITEMS

Anti-Inflammatory Herbs and Natural Sources

The concept of anti-inflammatory herbs is s very interesting one in the world of naturopathy and natural health. The reason why I gravitate towards them is that in the realm of inflammation and anti-inflammatory diets, they're a nice middle ground. Some people call for a total anti-inflammatory diet, eating only foods that promote the quelling of inflammation in the body. Others are on the Standard American Diet, eating a host of foods that are known to cause inflammation in the body and aggravate many disorders and conditions. Anti-inflammatory herbs are a nice in-between. Foods, in general, are said to be either pro-inflammatory or anti-inflammatory. As you might have guessed, foods that are pro-inflammatory will increase the amount of inflammation occurring in different parts of your body, will increase the pain associated with it, and may also increase your risk of having a chronic disease. Pro-inflammatory foods mostly are junk foods, sugars, fast foods, highly processed foods, and meats high in fat.

But that seems a bit excessive.That's why I love the idea of anti-inflammatory herbs.They're a nice middle ground in the world of inflammation, allowing you to stay healthy in that arena without putting too much of a focus on inflammation in general. Regularly eating some form of natural anti-inflammatory foods is key because it helps reduce the risk of things like arthritis and chronic autoimmune diseases. And because herbal concoctions are generally fairly strong, anti-inflammatory herbs are a great addition to meals, as well as in supplements.

Herbs generally have a wide variety of health benefits, and because inflammation is a somewhat complex process in the body, herbs can affect inflammation in different ways. Inflammation, when carried beyond reasonable limits, can become a type of autoimmune condition. It begins as negative stimuli cause white blood cells to activate and protect the area being negatively affected. Inflammation is necessary to the healing process, but chronic inflammation can cause lots of long term problems and is often excessive, like an allergic reaction.

Here are some of the best, most powerful anti-inflammatory herbs:

- Turmeric - Turmeric is a spice very common to most Indian foods. Though it has many other medicinal benefits, turmeric is a powerful anti-inflammatory herb. But it takes a bit of time to start working, so if you don't like the taste of turmeric, you might want to think about taking it in capsule form.

- Ginger - Ginger is also a spice that is used very often in Asian cooking. This spice also has a potent flavor and takes a bit of time to take effect within the body. Ginger is very versatile, being used in a range of both foods and drinks, so filling your diet with it shouldn't be too much of a challenge. You can drink ginger tea, ginger ale, use ginger in baked goods and spice meats with it.

- Omega 3 Essential Fatty Acids. Though these aren't technically herbs, omega three essential fatty acids are something that everyone needs more of in their diets. They're not only anti-inflammatory, but they also have a range of other medicinal benefits all across the body.

Liquorice - Liquorice is another herb that is very effective in the world of anti-inflammation. This too is a great herb to take because of its diversity. Liquorice is nice because it can be added to just about anything, like candy, tea, baked goods, vegetables, meats, and more, making it easy to get a high daily dose.

Mangosteen Juice - Mangosteen is a fruit native to Asia that has very powerful anti-inflammatory properties. Mangosteen juice is becoming more and more popular with persons who are suffering from the pain of arthritis, and mangosteen even has a very nice flavor. Many people substitute it for orange juice in their morning breakfast.

A few others worthy of note are:

- Pineapple juice

- Chamomile

- Black Seed Oil

- White Willow

- Red and Black Pepper

- St John's Wort

- Cilantro

- Cinnamon

- Garlic

- Cloves

Most diets are pretty profoundly deficient in anti-inflammatory herbs. I'm glad you're reading about what you can do to add more of them into your diet.

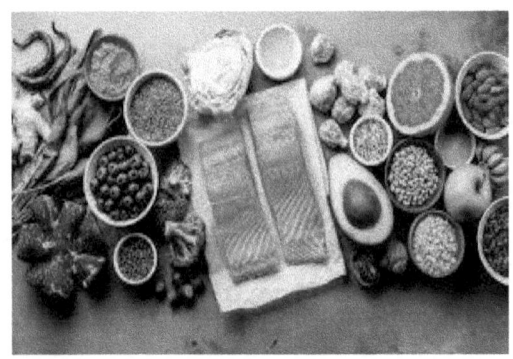

Natural Remedies - Anti Inflammatory Supplements

There are a lot of anti-inflammatory products on the market today. Unfortunately, many that you find over the counter are not very good for other parts of your body. For those with kidney or liver problems, an anti-inflammatory can be outright harmful. For those in good general health, over the use of these products can cause minor damage. Fortunately, there are many natural products that are very good at reducing swelling.

Bosweilla is a herb that is excellent at reducing joint inflammation associated with arthritis. A recommended dosage of 400 mg per day for arthritis is known to help reduce the discomfort associated with the disease. The origination of Bosweilla is in Africa. It has also been found in China as well as the Middle East. This herb works by blocking the inflammatory chemicals that are present in such diseases as osteoarthritis, atherosclerosis and other autoimmune diseases. It acts similarly as NSAIDS, although it does not block the cyclooxygenase-1 (COX-1), important in keeping the lining of the stomach healthy. It does block cyclooxygenase-2 (COX-2) which are a chemical that causes inflammation. To be effective, the Bosweilla should have at least 30% concentration of AKBA. This may take a bit of research to find.

Another supplement that all people should take, especially those affected by inflammation is Omega 3 fatty acids. There is a variety of Omega 3 products on the market. Searching out purified Omegas that do not have high levels of PCBs in them is very important. A bit of research on the internet can reveal which companies are steadfast in keeping their fish oils PCB free. The Omega 3s are a very necessary part of any diet and are especially helpful in controlling inflammatory issues.

Curcumin is found in the root of turmeric.It has a long-standing reputation of being used to treat stomach problems, chronic fatigue and arthritis.Recently, studies have shown that curcumin is also excellent as an anti-oxidant. Anti-oxidants are known to attack free radicals in the body. Free radicals are what causes pain and illness in the body.

Because inflammation happens for a variety of reasons in the body, such as infections, injury, or minor irritation or even a bug bite, choosing the correct herbal remedy is important. Not every herb that "fights inflammation" is going to be best for every type of swelling. Turmeric is good for arthritis and tendonitis. Bosweilla will dramatically help those who suffer from fibromyalgia symptoms. Other herbs, such as Arnica are great for reducing swelling found in bruises, or tooth and gum issues. White Willow Bark is an excellent headache remedy that many find great relief with.

So why all the fuss about using natural remedies instead of the over the counter stuff like ibuprofen?

Let's look at some of the side effects of these man-made products.Motrin is one of the most common anti-inflammatories on the market. Some of the side effects of this drug include cramping, gas and bloating. Those are quite common. That does not sound like something someone would want to experience if there was already inflammation and pain associated with that. Some of the more severe side effects include abdominal bleeding and ulcers in the gums and even depression or congestive heart failure. While these are rarer than the others, they are concerning, especially if someone is taking large amounts of ibuprofen for chronic pain.

It should also be noted that when taking Motrin or similar products, that the use of other products for swelling is not a good idea. The warning labels also state that people with kidney or liver issues should not take the Motrin. Diabetics should be aware of the sugar content in the ibuprofen products as well. With all of these warnings, side effects and cautions one has to consider if it is worth taking at all. Especially when there are some great natural remedies out there that are effective and don't have all the side effects.

With autoimmune disorders on the rise, so is the use of anti-inflammatory medication. There are so many possible side effects from over the counter products that one must consider the options. Natural health remedies such as Bosweilla and Omega 3 fatty acids and even the spice turmeric have no side effects, but have big benefits to the whole body. Fighting free radicals and bringing down inflammation is what will help bring the body back into balance. T

- ## *Top 4 Anti Inflammatory Supplements*

- Nature has given you a lot of resources to get you out of your inflammation, instead of taking toxic pharmaceutical drugs. Most of the traditional medicinal foods, herbs and spices used before centuries are still exploring today for making anti-inflammatory supplements.

- Let us see the top 4 anti-inflammatory supplements:

- Bioflavonoids: It is also called as flavones or

flavonoids. It is a class of five thousand plant chemicals that our bodies metabolize and offers strong anti-oxidant, anti-cancer, anti-allergenic and anti-inflammatory effects. Quercetin and epicatechin are some of the compounds that are included in Bioflavonoids. This bioflavonoid can be taken in supplemental form to prevent inflammation. Pine bark extract and grape seed extract are some of the natural extracts that are rich in bioflavonoid.

- Systemic Enzyme: This systemic enzyme offers something different from another natural anti-inflammatory. Compare to NSAID's that are usually used; the enzyme will not prevent our body from making all the protein chain CIC's like NSAID's do. It only dissolved the bad one, so the beneficial CIC's such as those that are keeping the kidneys to function and maintaining the lining of the intestines will remain in our body. It also reduces the inflammation all over your body, as well as the pain.

- Fish Oil: Omega-3 fatty acids are rich in fish oil. This reduces the production of the body's pro-inflammatory biochemical. People with rheumatoid arthritis have reduced their dosage of anti-inflammatory drugs after taking it. The effect of fish oil is in resonance with aspirin in inhibiting the synthesis of thromboxane A2 and leukotriene B4, which is highly inflammatory.

- Glucosamine - Chondroitin: Glucosamine sulfate and chondroitin sulfate are the essential building blocks of the cartilages. They help in repairing damaged tissues, and they are believed to delay the progression of joint inflammation. If you have this condition, consult with your health care provider about including this in your regular diet. These are the most recommended ones.

Omega-3 Anti-Inflammatory Supplements

What is an omega-3 natural anti-inflammatory

supplement and what benefits do they provide to those who take them regularly?

An omega-3 anti-inflammatory supplement is a natural nutritional supplement that has omega-3 fatty acids as its nutrient and benefits source, which is significant because omega-3 has very strong properties from being able to reduce and also inhibit inflammation.

Taking a supplement to manage inflammation is very beneficial because of the importance of keeping excess inflammation from building up in your body and becoming a chronic condition. If this happens, you will largely increase your risks for many different serious health problems, including an increased risk of heart disease and dying from a heart attack.

Additionally, joint problems and arthritis are a common condition, with millions of people suffering from their symptoms, and would very much benefit from an omega-3 anti-inflammatory supplement.

Where Does Omega-3 Come From?

Omega-3 is found in many plants and animals, but

there are a few things that are significant to note:

- Omega-3 are essential fatty acids, meaning that people need them but they are not made by our bodies, so the must be ingested through diet or supplements.

- Omega-3 is not a single fatty acid but a group of fatty acids.

- All omega-3 fatty acids do not have the same anti-inflammatory properties.

Keeping these things in mind, the omega-3 fatty acids that have the strongest anti-inflammatory benefits come from omega-3 DHA, with fish oil from cold water fish and green lipped mussels probably being the two best sources. On the other hand, omega-3 ALA, which is found in plants like flax, does not have inflammation reducing properties.

You especially hear about fish oil omega-3 supplements related to heart health. These are recommended by many heart health professionals, and the American Heart Association strongly recommends for people to increase the amount of fish in their diets - although this would be healthy and a good idea, getting the fish oil from a supplement will give a higher concentration source and further maximize the benefits.

For those with joint problems and arthritis, the green lipped mussel supplement omega-3 is likely more effective. Like the fish oil, the green lipped mussel will be a very good source for the omega-3 DHA anti-inflammatory, but the mussel supplements will also include omega-3 ETA. This fatty acid is a COX-2 inhibitor, which will help inhibit or keep inflammation from returning to your joints after it is reduced or eliminated.

So, when you start an omega-3 anti-inflammatory supplement, you will want to look at green lipped mussel supplements or fish oil supplements, with part of the decision being related to the specific reason for wanting a supplement to get rid of inflammation - but actually, if you will take both of these together you will receive synergistic benefits, and have the most effective anti-inflammatory alternative.

CHAPTER:-8

TIPS TO REDUCE INFLAMMATION
Knowledge on Reducing Inflammation in Your Body

Inflammation is one of the most common health problems that you could incur in your daily life. Such a health issue could occur owing to a wide variety of reasons. There are, however, various ways by which you can combat body inflammation. These contain eating health supplements and pursuing a proper and healthy diet. When you experience a health issue such as inflammation and you wish to know how you can get rid of it, there are some essential how to reduce inflammation in the body suggestions that you need to take into consideration.

One of the most important how to reduce inflammation in the body tips which you should take into consideration is eating food items that are rich in anti-oxidants. The antioxidants will improve digestion and circulation in your body. So if you consume the anti-oxidant rich food items, you will enjoy good body circulation and easy digestion. A few of the anti-oxidant rich food items that you should consume if you want to know how to get rid of inflammation are grapes, prunes, raspberries, blackberries, blueberries and strawberries. Another one of the how to reduce inflammation in the body tips which you should bear in mind is avoid processed foods. If you want to know how to reduce inflammation in the body, then you should also ensure that you avoid consuming the processed food items. This is because such food items do not have a high concentration of the anti-oxidants. These food items contain highly unhealthy food items like saturated fat, refined carbohydrates, trans-fat etc which can increase your body's inflammation issues. As a result, removing all the processed food items would be a good idea if you want to know how to get rid of inflammation in your body.

If you want to know how to get rid of inflammation in your body, then you should avoid drinking the sugar and carbonated drinks. Rather, one of the how to reduce inflammation in your body tips which you should consider is drinking plenty of water throughout the day. When you drink enough water during the day, your body stays well hydrated. When your body remains hydrated, digestion becomes very easy indeed. Green tea is a very good alternative to the carbonated drinks and sugary drinks along with water.

Exercising on a regular basis is also one of the most vital how to reduce the inflammation in your body tips that you should bear in mind. If you exercise for half an hour to one hour in the day, you will be able to lose weight quite naturally. This willresult in reduced inflammation. Thus, there are many how to do away with the inflammation tips that you can bear in mind for reducing your body inflammation. These how to dispense with the inflammation tips are known to be quite successful and are bound to ensure fruitful results if you follow them carefully.

Different Approaches to Reduce Inflammation and Pain

Are you tired of dealing with your chronic pain and

inflammation? Do you still wake up in the middle of the night screaming about the pain you've been suffering?

There are several ways you can do to help reduce inflammation and decrease the excruciating pain you're experiencing. Following these highly recommended tips and following these set of a healthy lifestyle, you can end your frustration with pain and live a happy and eventually, a pain-free life!

Lose some weight

If you're experiencing either an acute or chronic inflammation on the knee or hip area, consider to cut down your weight.

Carrying extra weight can only promote muscle and joint friction which greatly contributes to further pain and inflammation. Weight reduction is considered to decrease pain and stress to your muscles and joints if you're way over your ideal weight.

Do exercises on a daily basis

Moving your body especially your muscles and joints

on a regular basis can help reduce inflammation.

Exercising or doing isometric movements can relieve pain and muscle stiffness. If your muscles are not used, chances are, the affected muscles will atrophy and will constantly lead to weakness and immobility. Shake your mind and body and have a happy spirit to move along with your body!

Take time for adequate sleep and rest

Adequate rest is badly needed to take control of existing symptoms as well as a precautionary way to avoid excessive inflammation.It is a must to take minutes of rest every after your activity.

If you are experiencing chronic lower back pain, you need to condition yourself before doing any household chore and make sure to rest after each of your activity. This will help lessen inflicted pain on your lower back and eventually reduce inflammation and muscle strain.

Change your old eating habits

If you are still whining to eat fresh fruits and

vegetables in your midyear life, it's time to shake your head and wake up to reality. Living an unhealthy lifestyle won't guarantee you a prosperous and healthy body!

Change your old eating habits and stay away from foods that contain a large number of saturated fats and cholesterol. If you're not aiming to acquire musculoskeletal ailments such as rheumatoid arthritis, in the long run, it's time to stack your body and immune system with fresh vegetables that are high in fibre count.

Vegetables and garnishes such as leeks, garlic and onions are said to contain a huge amount of anti-inflammatory properties that can naturally reduce inflammation. Spice up your cooking and add an extra serving of fruits and vegetables every day.

Take in supplements and prescribed medications.

Taking in natural supplements and physician prescribed medications can help reduce and alleviate pain and inflammation. These drugs and natural supplements work effectively only if you follow a healthy diet, get adequate rest and do daily exercises. Medications alone would not cure your pain and its accompanying symptoms, you need to do something and start living a healthy lifestyle for you to completely get rid of inflammation. Act now and live a happy, well rested and healthy life.

Which Supplements Work to Decrease Inflammation?

You know lowering inflammation using standard methods can make you feel better, increase flexibility and experience less pain but do you know that anti-inflammatory herbs can make you feel better naturally? Decreasing pain, as well as irritation of inflammation, can elevate your mood, which in turn makes you want to move more, socialize more, and just do more. Without achy joints, you would love to take that walk with a friend, finish household chores, or continue other daily activities. Without irritable bowel syndrome, you may be less afraid to try the new restaurant you've been seeking.

Want to enjoy all the above things? But don't know

which anti-inflammatory herbs to choose, keep reading. In this part of this book, I have provided a few herbs that are effective and easy to find.

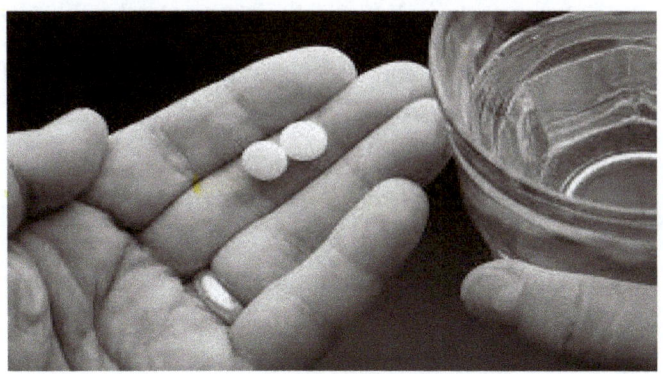

Ginger

By inhibiting the cyclooxygenase and lipoxygenase pathways, prostaglandin E2, thromboxane B2, and tumour necrosis factor, ginger decreases inflammation.

- It decreases pain in disorders such as osteoarthritis and rheumatoid arthritis.

- Ginger is antibacterial and antifungal. It is effective in decreasing fever.

- It aids with nausea, including the nausea of

pregnancy and nausea and vomiting of chemotherapy.

- It is also effective in decreasing the risk of heart and cardiovascular disease by increasing circulation and preventing the clotting of blood.

Turmeric/Curcumin

- Turmeric relieves indigestion by increasing digestive systems.

- It has hepatoprotective effects, which protect against liver damage.

- Decrease the risk of dementia and Alzheimer's disease and also helps with cognitive function.

- It reduces the inflammation and pain symptoms of rheumatoid arthritis.

- Turmeric works as a cancer preventative by inhibiting tumor promotion, inhibiting the growth of cancer cells and reducing their blood supply.

Boswellia

- It decreases inflammation in osteoarthritis, rheumatoid arthritis, tendonitis, bursitis, and general aches as well as pains.

- Boswellia may help decrease inflammation in asthma and allergies.

- It has antibacterial and antiviral properties.

- Boswellia is also reported to prevent cancer cell growth and help with programmed cancer cell death in colon cancer.

- It also protects against certain autoimmune diseases and their symptoms.

Blueberries

- These are high in antioxidants which protect cells from inflammation and oxidative stress.

- The anthocyanidins, which give blueberries their blue, red color, help keep blood vessels and capillaries strong.

- It helps stop the proliferation of cancer, and

enhance the antioxidants effects of vitamin C.

- It improves night vision and protects against muscular degeneration.

- Prevent aging of the brain due to free-radical damage, prevent dementia, and improve learning and motor skills.

These are only four anti-inflammatory herbs that are more effective on inflammation and other health issues. Other varieties of herbs that include flaxseeds, natural almonds, mushrooms and more choose the best herb(s) for your health problems and experience relief the natural way.

How to Reduce Pain and Inflammation Naturally

Having an inflammation tells you that something went wrong with your body.Common signs and symptoms of having an inflammation are warmth, redness, swollen body part and pain.

Sounds scary? There's no need to be afraid! There are natural ways on how you can reduce inflammation naturally following these do-it-yourself steps, precautions, and recommendations.

- Get an adequate amount of sleep - Sleeping is a good way to allow your entire body system to rest and allow time to heal from all the stresses your body concurred throughout the day. Sleeping hours may vary based on your activities of daily living, overall health, age and many other factors.

- Experts highly recommend that the ample amount of rest should range between 6 to 12 hours of sleep per day. Give up on your favorite late night show and go for a night of deep relaxing sleep instead.

- Get on your feet - Doing physical activities, exercise or range of motion (ROM) activities can help to naturally reduce muscle and joint inflammation.

- Engage in any activity or sport that you enjoy the most. It could be tennis, golf, ballroom dancing, yoga or any physical activity that pleases you. The bottom line is you need to move around, get your legs, feet, muscles and joints moving and have some fun.

- Stop smoking - Whoever said that smoking can bring a lot of benefit to your health?

- Smoking and nicotine found on cigarettes promotes hardening of the arteries and can increase CRP or C-reaction protein which is secreted by the liver and is a common response to inflammation.

- Quit smoking now, and it could help save you from lung and heart disease.

- Go for fruits and veggies - Craving for ice cream, pizza and fries? They may seem very delicious and enjoyable, but it is not highly recommended to eat these high saturated or fatty foods.

- Increasing your intake of fresh fruits and green leafy vegetables can help reduce inflammation to your body. Fruits and vegetables are known to possess high amounts of fiber and contain anti-inflammation properties which dramatically help reduce inflammation naturally.

- Introduce yourself to omega-3 fatty acids - Adding essential fatty acids or (EFAs) can help lessen chronic inflammation. Switch your cooking oil and go for olive oil when cooking. Opt for fish like salmon, sardines and tuna. They contain high levels of omega 3 which helps to lower inflammation and also promote a healthy heart.

Eating vegetables such as spinach, winter squash, broccoli and mangosteen, whole grains and nuts are also said to lower levels of inflammation.

Our modern diet may not contain sufficient amounts of EFA that can help decrease inflammation. Taking supplements that contain omega 3, high levels of antioxidants or Betalains may aid in reducing chronic inflammation.

It's always best to seek consultation with your physician to help you find the best supplements that can help you.

Remember not to only rely on these supplements but

make it a point to also get adequate sleep, increase your EFA intake, exercise moderately and live a healthy lifestyle.

CHAPTER:-9

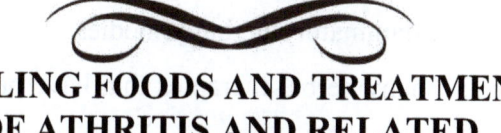

HEALING FOODS AND TREATMENT OF ATHRITIS AND RELATED DISEASES

Anti-Inflammatory Herbs - Herbal Remedies for Inflammation and Pain

Due to inflammation swelling, pain, redness or change in color of the skin is felt. But sometimes some internal inflammation can result giving rise to fever and other discomforts. The inflammatory response involves the activation of white blood cells that start releasing some chemicals such as cytokines and prostaglandins. Inflammation in some cases may be acute and chronic; some may often relapse depending on the severity of the disease. Inflammation is mostly treated by administering varied doses of corticosteroids that are effective in reducing and suppressing inflammation. Inflammation if not treated properly can aggravate some diseases causing much more problems, as in many cases it is difficult to predict an inflammatory response.

Few anti-inflammatory herbal remedies

There are many herbal therapies that have been tried through ages and have proven record in healing inflammation by treating the cause. Latest scientific researchers have given the final approval to opt for these herbal therapies than the OTC drugs.

- Turmeric is one of the common anti-inflammatory herbs that is widely used in Asian recipes in good amounts. It helps in reducing swelling, pain in arthritis, tendonitis, sprains and other autoimmune disorders. So the addition of extra turmeric in curries is beneficial in the long run! But this treatment is time-consuming, and it may test one's patience.

- Ginger is another herb which is popular for its anti-inflammatory properties and is used liberally in most Asian dishes. Taking ginger tea regularly in the morning relieves a lot of inflammation.

- Boswellin herb is very good inflammatory herb in treating fibromyalgia.

- White willow bark is another inflammatory herb that helps in reducing pain.

- Devil's claw works well in arthritis both in reducing inflammation and pain.

- Liquorice root is another popular anti-inflammatory herb, but its prolonged use may raise the blood pressure and cause potassium loss. So person suffering from hypertension must be cautious with its use.

- Arnica is another herb that is widely used in treating pains and bruises. It can be taken in regulated doses, or the mother tincture can be applied to the affected areas to reduce inflammation.

- St John's wort herb though used to treat depression also has some anti-inflammatory properties.

- Flax seed poultice is also very effective in treating bronchitis and reduces swellings in gouts and rheumatoid arthritis.

These herbs are very commonly used and are easily available. In sudden injuries, these can be applied immediately for some relief before consulting any doctor. These are cheap, and if applied properly one can avoid spending on painkillers and other drugs.

Arthritis Remedies and Herbal Treatments to Reduce Joint Pain and Inflammation

The term arthritis stands for a disorder affecting the joints and muscles around the joint. Every joint in the human body lies protected within a capsule. Cartilages occur at the boneheads of the two bones meeting at a joint. The joint cavity is filled with a lubricating fluid called synovial fluid. The cartilages at boneheads serve as cushioned pad resisting bone friction and allowing smooth movement of the bones. Due to factors like aging, obesity, previous history of bone damage or infection and heredity, cartilages often get weakened and start wearing out. This phenomenon characterized by the degeneration and loss of cartilage exposes bones to friction. The bones collide, get rubbed against each other and get eroded. Continuous erosion of bones due to friction may reduce the boneheads to spurs or osteophytes.

All this lead to joint inflammation and is named as arthritis. There are numerous types of arthritis, but the most widespread types are osteoarthritis, rheumatoid arthritis, and gout. Osteoarthritis is common among the elderly masses. In the case of osteoarthritis, aging triggers cartilage degeneration and bone friction. Rheumatoid arthritis attacks young people. It is an autoimmune disorder in which the immune system mistakenly attacks healthy tissues and organs. Gout is a condition which occurs due to crystallization of uric acid within the joint.

- Consumption of freshly grated ginger is a very good remedy for arthritis. Ginger prevents the production of inflammation-causing agents like prostaglandins and leukotrienes.

- Drinking tart cherry juice, and massaging affected joints with paraffin or hot vinegar before going to bed at night, can give some relief from joint pain.

- Homemade massage oil can be prepared by adding camphor or menthol to carrier oil. Camphor and menthol are very effective in easing muscle tightness, and soothing inflammatory conditions.

- Application of hot and cold compresses alternately can also bring down pain and stiffness.

- There are some herbs such as alfalfa, arnica, black cohosh, Boswellia, celery, ginseng, hops and rosemary that are widely used in the preparation of herbal supplements for arthritis. Many of these herbs possess anti-inflammatory and pain relieving properties that are helpful in reducing the pain and inflammation of the joints.

- Rumatone Gold oil and capsules have seasoned herbal ingredients and are very effective in treating arthritis. Massaging with rumatone gold oil helps a lot, for it penetrates into the body tissues easily, thereby reducing stiffness and improving mobility. When they are used in conjunction, provide quicker relief from the arthritis symptoms.

- Though, symptoms of arthritis are different for different types of arthritis. But some of its common symptoms are pain and stiffness in the joints, anaemia, colitis and deformed hands and feet.Usually after doing some exercise, the pain in the joints increases. In rheumatoid arthritis, the whole body is affected gradually.

There are different causes of arthritis. Some of its common causes are hormonal imbalance, physical and emotional stress, heredity and structural changes in the articular cartilage in the joints.

Arthritis can be treated in different ways to get an effective result. Many people go on changing their treatment plan as it suits them. But to find the best treatment for arthritis is a long process. The best goals of the treatment of arthritis are -

- To decrease the symptoms of arthritis.

- Maintain the function of the joint.

- To preserve mobility and range of motion.

- Prevent or minimize the damage and deformities in the joint.

- Slow progression of the disease.

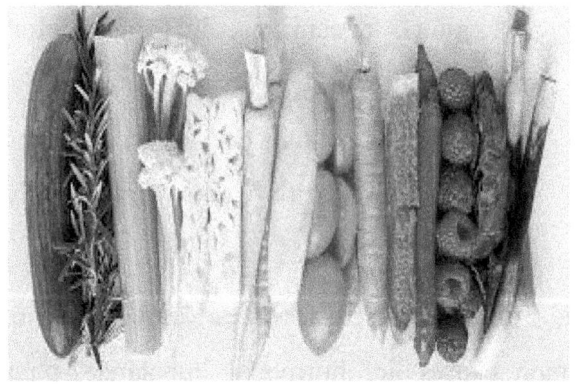

Different treatments of arthritis

- Treatment of arthritis through medication: It is considered to be the traditional treatment for arthritis. Doctors prescribe one or two medicines depending upon the severity of arthritis.

- Injections into a joint: Several types of

injections are there which can be given locally into the joint. For specific, painful joint local steroid injections can be used.

- Natural treatments: Nowadays most of the people are interested in natural treatments rather than going for traditional medications or joint injections. There are several options for natural treatment. They are known as alternative treatments. Though they are very popular but not fully endorsed for its safety and effectiveness.

- Complementary medicines: This type of treatment for arthritis is also very popular. It includes regular exercises, yoga, eating a nutritious diet, intake of fruits and green vegetables etc.

- Surgical options: Some people are left with no option rather than an opting surgical option. This is considered to be the last resort treatment option.

Herbal Cure for Leaky Gut Syndrome

The main way to deal with Leaky Gut Syndrome is through a proper and strict diet. It is important to get our body back to the best possible health condition. It is through avoiding foods or toxins that are causing the allergies so that the damaged intestinal lining will have a chance to heal and that the liver will have the energy and time it needs to detoxify the body.

It is possible to treat leaky gut naturally without the use of harsh prescribed medications.One way to do this is through the use of certain herbal remedies. Herbs have been used for years to cure a large range of ailments, and they can do the same these days.

A great herb to use is slippery elm. Slippery elm has been used as a balm to treat conditions such as skin inflammations, wounds, burns and boils. Because slippery elms have mucilage, a substance that turns into a gel when mixed with water, it can form a coating to soothe irritated throats, stomachs, and intestines. This does amazing things for leaky gut syndrome since the discomfort of intestinal lining is the cause of the condition. Plus, slippery elm also contains anti-oxidants which help to relieve this syndrome by reducing free radicals and relieving infections.

Chamomile tea also does amazing things for stomach problems. It is an efficient solution for reducing leaky gut symptoms such as bloating, gas, stomach cramps and pain. Drinking tea is also a natural way to relax. The symptoms of leaky gut syndrome intensify with stress or anxiety. One very efficient and natural treatment for aiding the reduction of this disease is to simply control the pressure or stress in your life.

Peppermint tea is also another herb that is used to relieve a variety of stomach problems including leaky gut syndrome. This tea relaxes the stomach and promotes the flow of bile. Plus, peppermint tea eliminates certain kinds of bacteria. When irritation of the bowels occurs with leaky gut, bacteria and harmful toxins can break free from the intestines and enter the bloodstream. A reduction in bacteria results in a decrease of the possibility of infection.

For many herbal specialists, the first choice for treating a huge range of problems is Echinacea. This herb is so highly effective that it has been used for malaria, scarlet fever, blood poisoning, and diphtheria. This herb helps to enhance the immune system, reduce swelling or inflammation, and it also possesses antioxidant qualities.

Another helpful herb to help reduce the symptoms of leaky gut is marshmallow root. This herb soothes the irritated mucous membranes of your digestive tract. It can be found at your local health food store or online and has been used for centuries to relieve just about all problems related to the swelling of the digestive tract.

When affected by Leaky Gut Syndrome, natural treatments are a useful option. Many times it is the excessive use of medications that worsen these symptoms. Antibiotics do not discriminate when eliminating off bacteria. Many times the good, beneficial bacteria that are normally found within intestines are affected and cannot do their job breaking up toxins. This can further aggravate the condition creating a severe pattern of symptoms.

Six Herbs to Treat Leaky Gut Syndrome

Is there possibly an all-natural treatment for Leaky Gut Syndrome, without the use of harsh prescription drugs? This could be done with the help of a few particular herbs. Today, as in centuries past, herbs are used to cure a multitude of different problems.

- SLIPPERY ELM - One wonderful herb to use is slippery elm. Slippery elm is an excellent treatment for such problems as skin inflammation, burns and boils. It is just as effective taken internally. Inflamed intestines, throats and belly are effortlessly soothed by slippery elm since it becomes gelatinous when mixed with water, letting it gently coat your insides. Since the irritation of the intestinal lining is what created this condition, this works fantastically for Leaky Gut Syndrome. This syndrome is also eased since slippery elm has antioxidants in it that relieves infection by eliminating free radicals.

- PEPPERMINT TEA - Another herb that helps get rid of a variety of digestive ailments, including Leaky Gut Syndrome, is peppermint tea. The intestines are calmed, and the flow of bile is promoted by this tea. And, peppermint tea helps eliminate specific types of bacterium. When irritation of the bowels happens with leaky gut, bacteria and toxins can escape from the intestines and enter the bloodstream. Reducing the bacteria also reduces the possibility of infection.

- CHAMOMILE TEA - Besides peppermint tea, another herbal tea named chamomile does superbly at treating gut issues. It works beautifully at easing Leaky Gut Syndrome symptoms such as bloating, excessive gas, cramping and belly pain. Drinking tea is also a natural way to relax. Symptoms of Leaky Gut Syndrome often exacerbate when one experiences excess anxiety or stress. Most people know that worrying and gut problems go hand in hand. An effective and conventional treatment for Leaky Gut Syndrome is to simply reduce your stress.

- MARSHMALLOW ROOT - Another

beneficial herb to decrease the symptoms of Leaky Gut Syndrome is marshmallow root. This herb soothes the irritated mucous membranes of your digestive tract. Used for centuries to relieve most problems with the belly, it might be found online or at a nearby health food store.

- ECHINACEA - Most herbalists would tell you that Echinacea may heal what ails you most of the time. It is so powerful it has even been used to treat Diphtheria, scarlet fever, blood poisoning and malaria. Performing like an antioxidant, reducing inflammation and strengthening the immune system are but a few of these herbs best qualities.

- GOLDENSEAL - Goldenseal is also favored by most herbalists. It is a potent herb, similar to Echinacea, and can be used to treat countless different problems while working particularly fast on intestinal conditions. It has been set on the endangered species list due to over-harvesting because it is so wildly popular.

- Organic remedies are such a valuable option when suffering from Leaky Gut Syndrome. This syndrome is commonly aggravated by the over utilisation of antibiotics. Antibiotics do not discriminate when killing off bacteria. This attack on the good bacteria commonly thriving inside the intestines does not allow them to do their natural job of eliminating allergens. This might further agitate the condition creating a harsh cycle of symptoms.

Leaky Gut Diet

Leaky gut deals with the small intestine. The small intestine has small pores that allow nutrients to pass into the bloodstream, such as valuable vitamins and minerals. When these pores become, enlarged other things can pass into the bloodstream also, such as; toxins, proteins, bad bacteria, and undigested particles. When bad things pass into the bloodstream, it can open the door for many things to go array with the health of your body and affect your quality of life.

What is Candida?

Candida is a buildup of yeast in the large intestine. A buildup of yeast in the large intestine can cause the pores in the small intestine to enlarge and allow unwanted things to pass into the bloodstream. These problems can also cause inflammation in the small and large intestine.

What is Chitosanase?

Chitosanase (by Bacillus coagulans) is a natural ingredient that addresses yeast in the gut. You will find this ingredient in a dietary supplement of probiotics. Not all probiotics have this natural ingredient; you will need to look for it. Just because it says it is a probiotic, does not mean that the ingredient "Chitosanase" is in it. You must look for this ingredient to be listed on the label.

Can Foods help with Leaky Gut?

Yes! Certain foods support healing because they are easy to digest and can help repair the lining of the intestines.

- Bone broth - Bone broth (made from scratch) provides important amino acids and minerals including proline, glycine and potassium that can help heal leaky gut and improve mineral deficiencies.

- Raw cultured dairy - Probiotic rich foods like deferring, amasai and yoghurt can help heal the gut by destroying bad bacteria.

- Fermented vegetables - Try to add fermented foods such as coconut, kefir, kvass, sauerkraut or kimchi. These fermented foods contain probiotics essential in helping to repair a leaky gut that works by balancing the pH in the stomach and small intestine.

- Steamed vegetables - Non-starchy vegetables that are cooked or steamed are easy to digest and are an essential part of the leaky gut diet.

- Healthy fats - Consuming healthy fats in

moderation like egg yolks, salmon, avocados, ghee and coconut oil are easy on the gut and promote healing.

- Fruits - Consuming 1-2 servings of fruit daily is good on a leaky gut diet. You can steam apples and pears to make homemade apple sauce or fruit sauce. Fruit is best consumed I the morning and not later on in the day and keep fruit intake in moderation.

Can Foods Cause Leaky Gut?

Yes! There are major foods in our daily diets that can attribute to Leaky Gut Syndrome and should be a serious consideration of control when planning our daily meals.

- Gluten - A gluten-free diet can help improve the symptoms of leaky gut. Gluten is the sticky protein found in most grain products including wheat and is difficult to digest unless it's been brought through a sourdough or sprouting process. On the leaky gut diet, you will want to avoid all foods that contain gluten and wheat products.

- Cows dairy - The protein in cow's dairy, called A1 casein, can trigger a similar reaction as gluten and therefore should be avoided. A1 casein may be 26 x more inflammatory than gluten.

- Sugar - Feeds yeast and bad bacteria that can damage the intestinal wall creating a leaky gut. If you are going to use a sweetener raw local honey is your best option, but even that should be consumed in moderation at 1 tbsp. Daily.

- Un-sprouted grains - Grains and soy when un-sprouted and unfermented contain phytic acid which can irritate the intestines causing leaky gut.

- GMO - Genetically modified organisms contain herbicides and pesticides that damage the gut lining. Studies out of the Journal of Environmental Sciences have found GMO foods destroy the probiotics in your gut and cause organ inflammation.

Gut health is very important to have healthy body organs and quality of life. A good way to tell if your gut is healthy is by monitoring your bowel movements.

Are you constipated? If your stool is rocky, then you are constipated!

Are your bowel movements regular? The answer is no if you only have one bowel movement a day.

Your bowels should move after you eat a meal. Your large intestine is as long as you are tall.That intestinal track should move every day. I do not mean empty out like cleaning for a colon test. I mean it should move, not sit still in your gut. When you have an overgrowth of yeast in your gut, this can cause many gut health problems. The purpose of your bowels is moving it to eliminate the toxins in your body. You want to rid your body of unwanted toxins as soon as possible; you do not want them sitting in your body causing unwanted health issues.

Did you know that your immune system is housed in

your gut?

If your gut is unhealthy and full of yeast, your autoimmune system is on vacation. When your autoimmune system is on vacation, it opens the door for autoimmune diseases to establish.

Let's name a few:

- Rheumatoid arthritis

- Lupus

- Fibromyalgia

CHAPTER:-10

A 15 DAY PERSONALIZED DIET PLAN

The anti-inflammatory diet has been very effective for many people and many different disorders. This is not a weight loss program, yet some people do lose weight while eating on this new and healthy path.

These are just general recommendations for the anti-inflammatory diet but please know that all health, as well as specific diets, are meant to be individualized, so take what you need and leave the rest behind. I advise you to work with a well-versed health care practitioner when making major shifts in your diet to assure you are getting the nutrients and nourishment you need. Feel free to contact me for more information or make an appointment if you would like to move forward in adding the anti-inflammatory diet into your life!

The Anti-Inflammatory Diet Basics

Tips for success

Try to eat organically grown foods as they reportedly have 2-5 time more nutrients and it will decrease exposure to pesticides.

There is no restriction on the amount of food you can eat, but as we have heard plenty of times, moderation is key, smaller portions more often throughout the day may work for you.

The foods listed are the only example of foods to eat.

Try to compose meals of approximately 40% carbohydrates, 30% proteins and 30% healthy fats.

Try to eat any one food no more than five times a week.

Plan your meals ahead of time to save time and stress later in the week.

Try to find a bunch of easy recipes that you enjoy to integrate into your cooking regime!

Antioxidant Rich Vegetables

Use mainly steamed vegetables as steaming improves the utilization or the availability of the nutrients, keeps the enzymes vital and is easier to digest

Use minimal raw veggies except as a salads

Include at least one green vegetable a meal

Fill half your plate each meal, actually eat as many servings as you'd like!

Eat a variety of any vegetables (except tomatoes and potatoes) that you can. It is best to try and eat mostly the lower carbohydrate (3-6%) vegetables.

3% - asparagus, bean sprouts, beet greens, broccoli, cabbage, cauliflower, celery, swiss chard, cucumber, endive, lettuce, mustard greens, radish, spinach, watercress

6% - string beans, beets, Brussel sprouts, chives, collards, eggplant, kale, kohlrabi, leeks, onions, parsley, red pepper, pumpkin, rutabagas, turnip, zucchini.

15% - artichoke, parsnip, green peas, squash, carrot

20% - yams

Add your favorite spices to enhance flavors

Eats lots of fermented veggies

Cold-water Fish

Poach, bake, steam or broil deep-sea ocean (wild rather than farmed fish) cod, haddock, halibut, mackerel, sardines, flounder, salmon is preferred
No shellfish
Aim for 3-4 servings a week.

Meats (from animals raised on their natural diets)

Eggs from pasture-raised hens
Meat from free-range or organically raised chicken, lamb, turkey.Bake, broil or stream.

Fruits

Eat only 1 or 2 pieces of practically any fruit (except citrus)
Like the vegetables, try to eat mostly the low carbohydrate fruits for example:
3% - cantaloupe, rhubarb, strawberries, melons
6% - apricot, blackberries, cranberries, papaya, peach, plum, raspberries, kiwi
15% - apple, blueberries, cherries, grapes, mango,

pear, pineapple, pomegranate

20+% - banana, figs, prunes, and dried fruit.

Avoid juice and dried fruits as they contain high amounts of sugar.

Limit to 2-3 servings a day

Herbs and Spices

Cinnamon, Turmeric, ginger, garlic, rosemary and thyme are all great herbs to help reduce inflammation!

To add a delightful flavour to your food, add whatever spices you enjoy!

Beverages

Drink a minimum of 6-8 glasses of clean and pure water every day

A few drops of chlorophyll will add a pleasant taste, and help build blood

No distilled water

Homemade Broth

Herbal tea

Kombucha/ fermented beverages

Day 1 Meal Plan

Breakfast: Tea of choice, oatmeal made with soy milk and topped with blueberries, ground flaxseeds, half a banana and a sprinkling of cinnamon

Lunch: Spinach salad with cherry tomatoes and grilled salmon, with an extra-virgin olive oil and lemon juice dressing

Dinner: A chickpea and vegetable curry (try sweet potato, peas, spinach, cauliflower, Asian mushrooms, turmeric etc.) with brown rice

Day 2 Meal Plan

Breakfast: One omega-3 enriched organic egg, poached, on a slice of wholegrain toast and an apple

Lunch: Homemade miso soup with soba noodles, peas, mushrooms and green onion; a salad with avocado, mango, mixed greens, cherry tomato and a lime and olive oil vinaigrette

Dinner: Wholegrain pasta – cooked al dente – with kale, hemp & flaxseed oil

Day 3 Meal Plan

Breakfast: Smoothie with leafy greens of your choice, a banana, a tablespoon of seeds (hemp, flax or chia), pinch of cinnamon and non-dairy milk or water

Lunch: Leftover pesto pasta from Day Two; a pear or serving of melon

Dinner: Thai-style steamed trout made with ginger, chilli, lime, garlic and soy sauce, served with broccoli and a baked sweet potato

Day 4 Meal Plan

Breakfast: Chia pudding made with soymilk, cinnamon and a banana

Lunch: Vegetable and lentil soup; an orange

Dinner: Chicken fajitas with one organic chicken breast, mixed vegetables and spices topped with salsa, half an avocado and served in 1 to 2 wholegrain tortilla wraps

Day 5 Meal Plan

Breakfast: Same smoothie as Day Three

Lunch: Chopped power salad with baked tofu and

almond-miso dressing served with a wholegrain pita bread

Dinner: Pan-seared fish with shiitake mushrooms served with sautéed green vegetables and quinoa

Day 6 Meal Plan

Breakfast: Overnight oats made with soy milk or yoghurt, topped with nuts, shredded coconut and fresh fruit; green tea with fresh ginger

Lunch: Lemon and herb sardine salad; an apple

Dinner: Sweet potato, black bean and rice burger in a wholegrain bun, with sliced avocado and a green salad; followed by tea of your choice

Day 7 Meal Plan

Breakfast: Coconut Turmeric Quinoa Porridge

Lunch: Lettuce 'Tacos' with Chipotle Chicken

Dinner: Turmeric Cauliflower Curry

Day 8 Meal Plan

Breakfast: Quick Carrot Rice Breakfast Nasi Goreng

Lunch: Avocado Tuna Salad

Dinner: Baked Honey Cilantro Lime Salmon

Day 9 Meal Plan

Breakfast: Pineapple Ginger Turmeric Protein Smoothie

Lunch: Thai Cucumber Noodle Salad

Dinner: Chili Lime Salmon Tacos with Mango Salsa

Day 10 Meal Plan

Breakfast: Golden Milk Chia Pudding

Lunch: Cajun Garlic Shrimp Noodle Bowls |

Dinner: Zucchini Fritters with Avocado Dill Dip

Day 11 Meal Plan

Breakfast: Poached eggs served with spinach, avocado, shiitake mushrooms and barley

Lunch: Rocket, tomato, cucumber and tuna salad served with brown rice

Dinner: Steak, grilled or lightly pan-fried, with cannellini bean mash and sautéed greens

Day 12 Meal Plan

Breakfast: Beets and Berries Overnight Oats

Lunch: Shrimp and Avocado Salad with Miso

Dressing

Dinner: Turmeric Miso Soup with Ginger, Garlic and Tofu

Day 13 Meal Plan

Breakfast: Black beans cooked with canned chopped tomatoes and a few herbs served with wholegrain toast

Lunch: Salad of chickpeas, lettuce and tomato topped with roast vegetables

Dinner: Pan-fried snapper served with sautéed spinach and herbed rice salad

Day 14 Meal Plan

Breakfast: Green smoothie made from any two servings of green vegetables and one serve of fruit

Lunch: A generous serving of sauerkraut topped with fresh salmon. Add half an avocado and salad vegetables of your choice, drizzled with olive oil

Dinner: Chinese cabbage, tofu ginger and chilli stir-fry served with brown rice

Day 15 Meal plan

Breakfast: Homemade granola made from oats, seeds and nuts with berries and Greek-style yoghurt

Lunch: Soup of lentils and mixed vegetables

Dinner: Grilled salmon, spread with a turmeric and ginger paste, served with beetroot and lentil salad